EDEXCEL
Health and Social Care
for GCSE

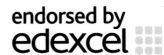
endorsed by
edexcel

EDEXCEL
Health and Social Care
for GCSE

Hilary Thomson and Sylvia Aslangul

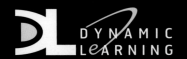
DL DYNAMIC LEARNING

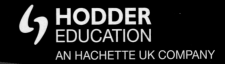
HODDER EDUCATION
AN HACHETTE UK COMPANY

Orders: please contact Bookpoint Ltd, 130 Milton Park, Abingdon, Oxon OX14 4SB. Telephone: (44) 01235 827720. Fax: (44) 01235 400454. Lines are open from 9.00–5.00, Monday to Saturday, with a 24-hour message answering service. You can also order through our website www.hoddereducation.co.uk

If you have any comments to make about this, or any of our other titles, please send them to educationenquiries@hodder.co.uk

British Library Cataloguing in Publication Data

A catalogue record for this title is available from the British Library

ISBN: 978 0 340 975 091

First Edition Published 2009

Impression number   10 9 8 7 6 5 4 3 2 1

Year   2012, 2011, 2010, 2009

Hachette UK's policy is to use papers that are natural, renewable and recyclable products and made from wood grown in sustainable forests. The logging and manufacturing processes are expected to conform to the environmental regulations of the country of origin.

Cover photo © Corbis/Photolibrary Group Ltd

Illustrations by Kate Nardoni of Cactus Design & Illustration Ltd

Typeset by Servis Filmsetting Ltd, Stockport, Cheshire

Printed in Italy for Hodder Education, an Hachette UK Company, 338 Euston Road, London NW1 3BH

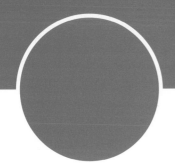

INTRODUCTION

This book has been written to support students who are studying for the Edexcel GCSE in Health and Social Care. Those who are taking the Single Award will cover Unit 1 and Unit 2. Those who are taking the Double Award will cover all 4 units. This GCSE in Health and Social Care uses the course structure designed by Edexcel. The book is developed to cover the 4 GCSE Units:

Unit 1 Understanding Personal Development and Relationships
Unit 2 Exploring Health, Social Care and Early Years Provision
Unit 3 Promoting Health and Wellbeing
Unit 4 Health, Social Care and Early Years in Practice

This book has been developed to cover each of these units in detail. Headings are designed to make it easy to follow the content of each unit. Throughout the book, there are activities and discussion points that can help students apply their learning to real life situations linked to health and social care issues.

Assessment

Unit 1 is assessed through a one written examination paper, with a total of 70 marks lasting one hour and 15 minutes.
The paper consists of 15 multiple choice questions and a series of questions based on case studies and short scenarios.
Unit 2 is internally assessed through one Edexcel-set task to be completed under controlled conditions. It will be internally assessed and externally moderated and is marked out of 50
Unit 3 is assessed internally through one Edexcel-set task based on pre-release material. This is to be completed under controlled conditions. It will be internally assessed and externally moderated and is marked out of 50
Unit 4 is assessed externally by one written examination paper with a total of 70 marks, lasting one hour and 15 minutes. The paper consists of three compulsory questions based on case studies and short scenarios.

Detailed guidance for internal and external assessment can be found on the Edexcel website www.edexcel.org.uk

The Edexcel GCSE in Health and Social Care assesses particular skill areas:

A01 Students will demonstrate their ability to recall, select and communicate their knowledge and understanding of health and social care in a range of contexts
A02 (i) Students will demonstrate their ability to plan and carry out investigations and tasks
A02 (ii) Students will demonstrate their ability to apply skills, knowledge and understanding in a variety of contexts
AO3 Students will show evidence of analysis and evaluation

Special features of this book

Throughout the book there are a number of features that are designed to encourage students to discuss issues related to health and social care. Students will develop their skills in the following areas in preparation for the assessment

- analysing data
- linking discussion of theory to health and social care practice
- identifying trends in practice
- finding out relevant information
- presenting information in a range of formats
- revising key aspects of the qualification
- preparing for the assessment
- taking part in discussions

Case Studies

The use of case studies throughout the book encourages students to apply the knowledge they have gained to actual examples in health and social care. Many students are unable to have work experience in health and social care, so case studies are a way of introducing them to relevant examples that occur in a range of health, social care and early years settings.

Key terms

Throughout the book there are key terms that are highlighted in the text and the authors give a brief explanation of how these terms may be used

Glossary

This book contains a full glossary at the end of the book and, to provide fast reference for key terms, a shortened glossary of those terms used within chapters.

The authors are experienced teachers and have written numerous Health and Social Care textbooks.

1 Understanding Personal Development and Relationships

Human growth and development

How do individuals grow and develop during each life stage?

- Growth is an increase in physical size (mass and height).
- Development is the process of the gain, and increase in complexity, of new skills, abilities and emotions.

Milestones, or norms, show what most children can do at a particular age. However, it is important to remember that, although using norms helps us understand patterns of development, each child will, of course, develop in their own unique way and there will be wide variation between individuals. Keep this in mind when using the development tables below.

Throughout a person's life, growth and development should be considered under the following headings:

- Physical (concerned with functioning of the body)
- Intellectual (concerned with ability to think and understand)
- Emotional (concerned with ability to recognise and express feelings appropriately)
- Social (concerned with ability to relate to others and form relationships).

(Remembering the word 'pies' should help you learn these headings (see Figure 1.1).

Each of these types of development is described in detail below.

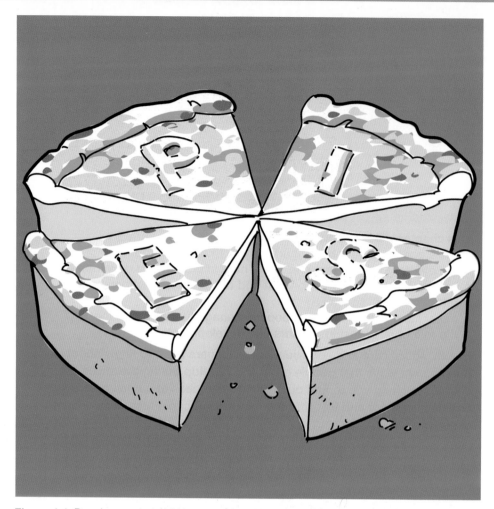

Figure 1.1 Development should be considered under the headings

The different life stages

Growth and development takes place during each of the six main life stages (see Figure 1.2).

Life stage	Age span (years)
Infancy	0–2
Early childhood	3–8
Adolescence	9–18
Early adulthood	19–45
Middle adulthood	46–65
Later adulthood	65+

Table 1.1 Six main life stages

For the first eight weeks after fertilisation, a human is known as an embryo. After eight weeks and before birth, it is known as a foetus.

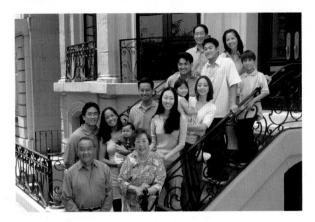

Figure 1.2 Different life stages

Physical Growth and Development

Growth

Growth in infancy

There are various ways of measuring the growth of a baby. The three measurements most commonly made are:

- mass (usually referred to as weight)
- length
- head circumference.

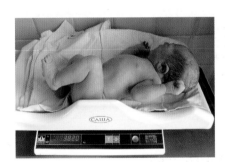

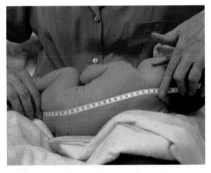

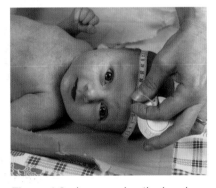

Figure 1.3 a) weighing a baby

Figure 1.3 b) measuring the length of a baby

Figure 1.3 c) measuring the head circumference of a baby

A newborn baby, on average:

- weighs 3.5 kg
- has a length of about 50 cm
- has a head circumference of about 35 cm.

Boys are, on average, about 100 g heavier than girls, and slightly longer. A baby grows very quickly in the first two years of life. Typically, a baby will grow 25–30 cm and triple in body weight in the first year.

The body parts of a baby do not all grow at the same rate. For example, in the first year:

- the legs and arms grow at a faster rate than the rest of the body
- the head grows at a slower rate than the rest of the body.

Figure 1.4 shows how the different growth rates of the various parts of the body lead to changes in the proportions of the body.

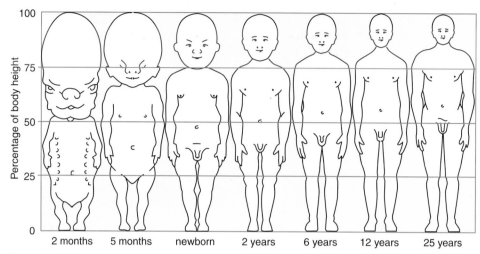

Figure 1.4 The proportions of the body change throughout life

ACTIVITY

1. Figure 1.5 shows the average weights, lengths and head circumferences of boy babies

Look at this and work out how long it takes for an average boy baby to double its birth weight. (Give your answer to the nearest month.)

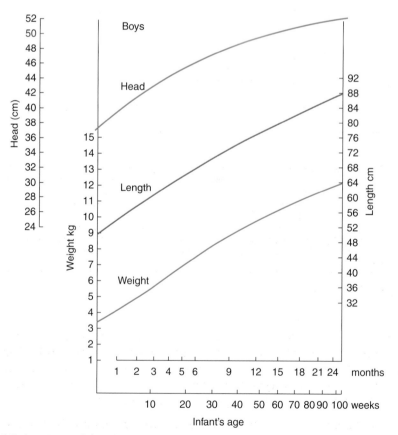

Figure 1.5 Average weights, lengths and head circumferences of boy babies

Percentile charts

These are used to compare babies' growth with the rest of the population. Look at the percentile chart in Figure 1.6.

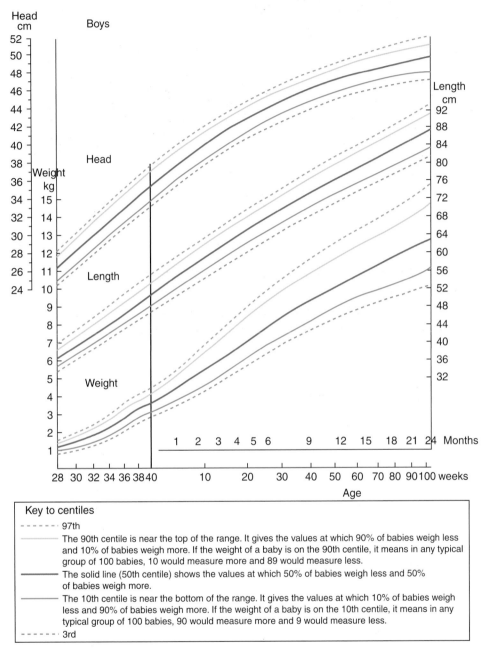

Key to centiles

- - - - - - 97th

———— The 90th centile is near the top of the range. It gives the values at which 90% of babies weigh less and 10% of babies weigh more. If the weight of a baby is on the 90th centile, it means in any typical group of 100 babies, 10 would measure more and 89 would measure less.

———— The solid line (50th centile) shows the values at which 50% of babies weigh less and 50% of babies weigh more.

———— The 10th centile is near the bottom of the range. It gives the values at which 10% of babies weigh less and 90% of babies weigh more. If the weight of a baby is on the 10th centile, it means in any typical group of 100 babies, 90 would measure more and 9 would measure less.

- - - - - - 3rd

Figure 1.6 Percentile chart

Growth in early childhood

By the time a child is 3-years-old, their weight is generally about four times their birth weight. Figure 1.7 shows growth rate between the ages of 2 and 9. During this time growth takes place at a fairly constant rate, and at a slower rate than the growth between 0–2 years. Typically, a child will gain 5–8 cm in height and about 3 kg in body weight per year from age three to adolescence.

The skull and brain have usually reached adult size by the time the child is about 5-years-old, but after this the child's appearance changes as the upper

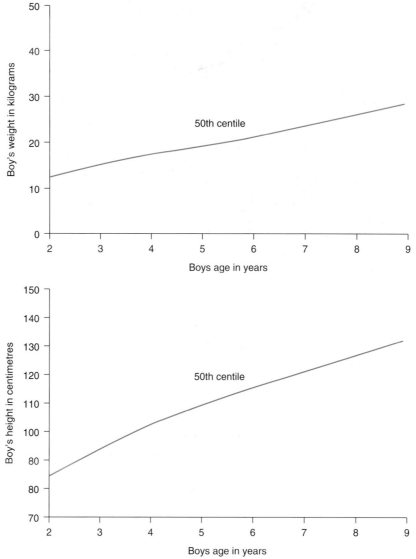

Figure 1.7 a) Average weights of boys (2–9 years);
b) Average heights of boys (2–9 years)

and lower jaws grow rapidly, and the first set of teeth are replaced by the permanent teeth.

Growth in adolescence

In adolescence there is a sudden increase in growth rate and maturity. This produces an adult who would be able to produce and care for young.

Adolescence starts with puberty, which is the time during which secondary sexual characteristics develop (see Figure 1.8). Puberty usually starts at about age 10 in girls, and 12 in boys. By their late teens the changes are usually complete.

The changes are bought about by sex hormones. Oestrogen and progesterone cause the changes in females, and testosterone in males.

The increase in growth rate in adolescence is known as the second growth spurt. Height may increase by 8–16cm per year.

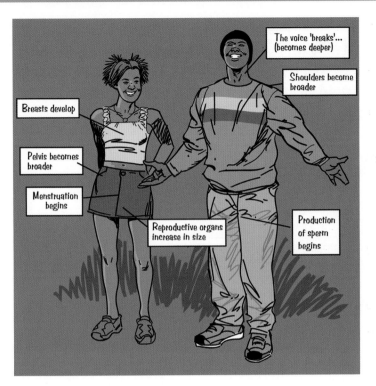

Figure 1.8 Secondary sexual characteristics

The second growth spurt is different in males and females:

- In girls the growth spurt usually occurs between about 10 and 14 years, but in boys it is usually between about 12 and 16-years-of-age.
- In boys the growth spurt lasts longer than in girls, which means men are generally larger than women.

Growth in early and middle adulthood

By the end of adolescence the body is physically and sexually mature. Although growth no longer takes place after about 18–20 years of age, physical changes to the body continue as the body ages.

The menopause occurs in women, usually between about 45 and 55. After this they do not produce eggs, which means they can no longer become pregnant. Men, however, can produce sperm and can father children into old age.

Growth in later adulthood

Figure 1.9 shows how the main body systems deteriorate with age. Despite these changes, the ageing process can be approached with a positive attitude. Improved health care (among other factors) has increased life expectancy and the quality of life in old age. Their wealth of experience allows elderly people to make valuable contributions. It is unfortunate that some young people portray all older people as being ready for the nursing home by the time they are 65!

Physical development

Physical development is the way in which the body increases in skills and complexity of performance. The physical skills which develop throughout life can be divided into two main areas: gross motor skills and fine motor skills (see Figure 1.10).

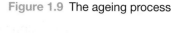

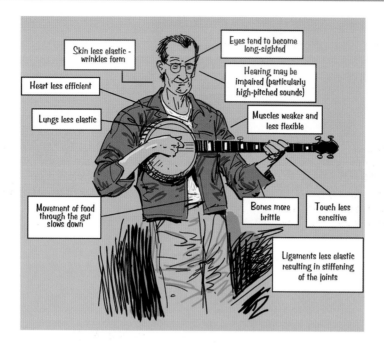

Figure 1.9 The ageing process

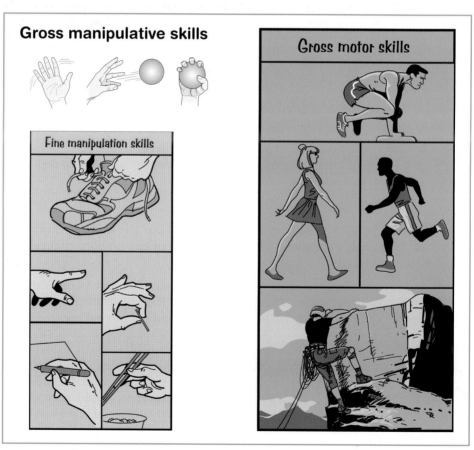

Figure 1.10 The main areas of physical development

- **Gross motor skills** use the large muscles of the body and involve movement of the whole body, (for example, walking and climbing).
- **Fine motor skills** may involve single limb movements (for example, throwing) or precise use of the hands and fingers (for example, drawing, using a keyboard or doing up a button).

Physical development in infancy

Table 1.2 shows the development of both gross motor skills and fine motor skills in infancy.

Age	Gross motor skills	Fine motor skills
Birth–4 weeks	• Lies on back with head to one side • If placed on front turns head to one side • By one month can lift head	• Will turn head towards light and stares at objects • Stares at carer's face • Hands usually tightly closed
4–8 weeks	• Can turn from side to side on back • Can lift head briefly when lying face down • Arm and leg movements jerky and uncontrolled.	• Shows interest and excitement by facial expressions • Opens hand to grab finger
8–12 weeks	• Can lift head and supported by forearms when laying face down • Kicks legs vigorously • Can wave arms and bring hands together	• Moves head to follow person • Plays with fingers • Holds rattle for short time
4–5 months	• Good head control • Beginning to sit with support • Can roll from back to side • Reaches for objects when on back • Plays with feet	• Beginning to use palmer grasp • Transfers objects from hand to hand • Puts object in mouth
6–9 months	• Can roll from front to back • May attempt to crawl • Can sit without support • May 'cruise' around furniture and even stand	• Beginning to use pincer grip

Table 1.2 Physical development in infancy (0–2 years)

Age	Gross motor skills	Fine motor skills
9–12 months	● Baby mobile: crawling, bear-walking, bottom shuffling or even walking ● Sits up on own and leans forward to pick things up ● May crawl upstairs	● Points with one finger ● Claps hands ● Drops toys deliberately ● Holds spoon and finger food
15 months	● Baby walks unsteadily ● Climbs up stairs ● Kneels without support	● Holds crayons in palmar grasp ● Turns several pages of a book at once ● Shows preference to one hand but uses either
18 months	● Walks confidently ● Carries things ● Climbs ● Comes down stairs backwards, or on tummy	● Threads large bead ● Builds tower of three or more bricks ● Scribbles

Table 1.2 (continued)

Age	Gross motor skills	Fine motor skills
2 years	● Runs ● Walks up and down stairs ● Kicks a ball	● Draws circles lines and dots with preferred hand ● Builds a tower of six or seven bricks ● Turns a single page of a book

Table 1.2 (continued)

Physical development in childhood

Table 1.3 shows the development of both gross motor skills and fine motor skills (manipulative skills) in childhood.

Age	Gross motor skills	Fine motor skills
3 years	● Jumps from low step ● Walks backwards ● Stands on tip toes and one foot ● Pedals tricycle	● Builds tower of nine or ten bricks ● Holds pencil correctly with pincer grip ● Paints with large brush
4 years	● May walk along a line ● Run up and down stairs ● Stands on one leg, jumps up and down	● Catch, kick, throw and bounce ball ● Builds a tower of ten or more bricks ● Draws a circle and a cross ● Threads small beads on lace
5 years	● Uses play equipment (e.g. slides, climbing frames and swings) ● Hops ● Skips	● May thread large-eyed needle and stitch ● Draws a person with face ● Copies square and triangle ● Buttons clothes

Table 1.3 Physical development in early childhood (ages 3–8 years)

Age	Gross motor skills	Fine motor skills
6 and 7 years	● Increased agility, co-ordination and balance ● Rides bicycle	● Draws a person in detail ● Writes letters of the alphabet ● Catches a ball with one hand from distance of a metre ● Ties laces
8 years	● Continued increased agility, co-ordination and balance	● Writing continues to improve

Table 1.3 (continued)

Physical development in adolescence, adulthood, old age

By the time the nervous system is fully developed, all the main developmental milestones will have been reached. However, even in later life, people may learn new gross and fine motor skills.

ACTIVITY

1. Read below the list of skills that may be acquired in adulthood. Which are gross motor skills and which are fine motor skills?
   ● Embroidery
   ● Skiing
   ● Playing the flute
   ● Horse riding.
2. Can you think of any physical skills that you have learnt since childhood?

Intellectual/cognitive development including language development

Intellectual/cognitive development refers to the development of the parts of the brain concerned with:

- perception (absorbing information about the environment through the senses of sight, hearing, touch, smell and taste)
- acquiring knowledge
- reasoning
- understanding.

Nearly every brain cell a person has is present at their birth. During childhood the brain grows very quickly. By the age of one year, the baby's brain is already three-quarters of its adult size and rapid development continues until middle childhood.

Intellectual/cognitive development in old age

In old age there may be changes in memory, but only in certain aspects. Long-established skills, such as money management, playing a musical instrument or gardening, remain unaffected by old age. The memory for names and everyday activities, however, may be affected. Sometimes, an old person may find it difficult to distinguish between a real and an imagined event. For example, an elderly person may believe they have turned the gas off, when in reality they have only *thought* about turning it off.

The ability to recall events from the distant past improves slightly into middle age, and by the age of 60 shows only a slight decline.

Emotional maturity across the life stages

Emotional maturity involves the development of self-image and identity and the ways in which individuals make sense of themselves and of the feelings they have towards other people.

Table 1. 6 shows how emotional maturity develops across the life stages.

As we can see from Table 1.6, there are key stages in our lives which affect our emotional development. Developing a 'sense of self 'continues throughout our lives, and if we feel supported by others and we also feel that we have some purpose in life, we can experience all life stages in a positive way.

There are some key terms in the table that we need to discuss.

> **KEY TERM**
>
> **Bonding** – is making an emotional attachment to a person and is usually to do with the close relationship of a baby to its mother.

Life Stage	Development
Infancy	
1–2 months	Infants recognise and react to other people and build emotional attachments with their parents and carers
By 1-year-old	Infants can recognise and react to emotional expressions of happiness, distress and anger. They may reflect the emotions shown to them by their parents or carers
By 2-years-old	Infants have a sense of self and of their gender as male or female. The child forms an emotional bond with their parents
Early childhood	From two and a half years children use their imagination and copy what they see others doing – such as mother caring for baby. Play develops. They develop a sense of self and can describe themselves in detail by the age of 8
Adolescence 9–18 years	During this time adolescents can say what makes them happy or sad, and why they like certain people. They begin to compare themselves with others in looks and skills. Friends become more important than family; friends influence their 'self-concept'. The physical changes adolescents go through can make them unhappy and unsure of themselves and they can be moody, angry and 'difficult'. Friends are their main social support. They often develop beliefs which are different from those of their parents – vegetarianism, animal rights, religion; this is seen as 'rebelling'. They can also be very idealistic
Early adulthood 19–45 years	Self-concept is still developing through certain events such as marriage or a stable partnership, or a successful career path. This age group can make decisions in family (buying a house) and work life (taking a new job). The twenties can be seen as a stressful time, as it is a 'settling down' period before a more stable life develops, as a result of deciding upon lifestyle, career and partnerships

Table 1.6 How emotional maturity develops across the life stages

Life Stage	Development
Middle adulthood 46–65 years	At this stage adults should have developed a strong sense of 'self'. They may have to deal with family break-ups, unemployment and the death of close family members. These events may have a positive or a negative effect on a person's emotional development. Success in work, or in the family, can increase a person's self-concept. On the other hand, women who have had a bad experience of the menopause, or of their children leaving home, can develop a negative self-concept
Later Adulthood 66 years+	At this stage in life, long-term illness may affect someone's self-concept in a negative way. Older adults who have ceased working and have limited social contact may feel that they are 'invisible' in today's society where the emphasis is on youthfulness and staying young. Loss of self-esteem can affect both men and women who have retired after a successful career. However, if they keep active and maintain social contact they could find pleasure in their later lives

Table 1.6 (continued)

Bowlby (1953) felt that separation of a baby from its mother could damage the child emotionally. Many mothers returning to work feel anxious about harming their baby by leaving them with another carer, but later researchers felt that if the bond between mother and child is strong, separation will not harm the child emotionally.

Self-concept across the life stages

Everyone has a view of themselves known as the self-concept (see Figure 1.11). This is based upon the beliefs that they have of themselves as a person, and also on what other people think about them.

Figure 1.11 shows the factors that affect a person's self-concept.

We will look at some of these factors in turn.

Age

We can see that our self-concept develops throughout the life course (see Table 1.6). In order for the concept of 'self' to develop, you first have to see yourself as a separate physical being. As we age we use information from others to confirm our view of ourselves.

Appearance

We are influenced in our self-concept by the opinion of others and by how we compare ourselves with media images. People tend to be more sensitive to this influence on their self-concept in their adolescence and adult lives. If you look at magazines or papers you can see that certain images of men and women are promoted. Women are supposed to be slim, well-dressed and use make-up. Men are supposed to have athletic bodies and be well-groomed. Role models such as footballers or fashion models show the aspirations of many young people. As we get older, appearance becomes less important. This could be because of other changes in our lives, such as parenthood, family commitments or more self-confidence in our feelings about ourselves. Experiments have been carried out where people have changed their appearance and they noticed a change in the way other people reacted to them – this showed how other people's reactions affect our self-image. One actress wore a 'fat suit' and found that people's attitudes were hostile and unfriendly. Another actress made herself up to look

KEY TERM

Role model – an example of behaviour or achieved status in society that is seen as good.

Self-concept has several components:

- **Self-image** – how you see yourself and what you know about yourself. This is affected according to your cultural background. In most Western societies, people tend to focus on their individual personality traits. In Japanese and other cultures, people tend to describe themselves as part of a social group.

- **Ideal self** – refers to the person you would like to be. We can be influenced by the media, parents and teachers.

- **Self-esteem** – refers to how you feel about yourself and judge yourself. How much do we like the kind of person we are? Do we accept ourselves as we are?

Figure 1.11 (a)

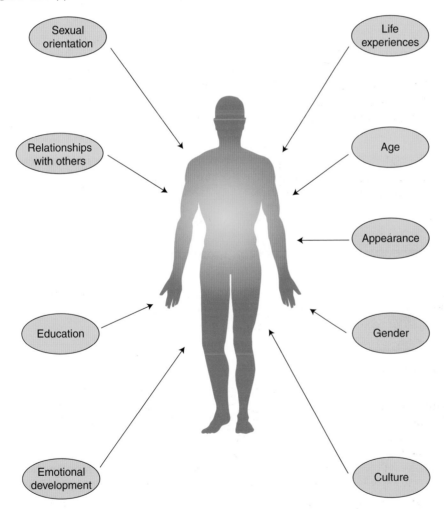

1. Age
2. Appearance
3. Gender
4. Culture
5. Emotional development
6. Education
7. Relationships with others
8. Sexual orientation
9. Life experiences

Figure 1.11 (b) Factors affecting a person's self-concept

like an old lady and found that shop assistants ignored her in shops, and people generally tended to avoid responding to her. A white actor made his skin darker and changed his style of dress, making it more casual and 'hip hop', and found that white youths were aggressive towards him. A student on a psychology course decided to test how helpful people would be to him if he was in a wheelchair in a busy shopping area. He found that he was ignored or any comments were made to his friend, who was pushing the wheelchair.

We can see from these examples that appearance can make a difference to the reactions of others to you, and in turn this can affect your self-concept.

Gender

When a baby is born, it is biologically identified as either male (having a penis) or female (having a vagina). Gender refers to the psychological or social aspects we develop as we grow up. Gender identity is a clear understanding of ourselves as either male or female, and as part of our development we take on the expected social roles of males and females in our society. Boys play with action figures and are boisterous in play. Girls enjoy playing with dolls and are quieter. These are the gender stereotypes that we are expected to conform to.

Children know whether they are boys or girls by the age of 2. Their play and choice of friends reflects their gender identity. Up to the age of 7, boys and girls play with either sex, but after this age they prefer to play with members of their own sex. Gender identity is reinforced through the media. Television adverts show traditional toys for boys and girls in the period before Christmas. Parents are also influential in promoting gender differences.

Expectations of others based on gender, can lead to problems if girls want to follow non-traditional female jobs, such as becoming car mechanics or plumbers. It can also be difficult for boys who want to be nurses or carers of family members. Ann Oakley did some studies when she interviewed housewives (Housewife, 1974). She was interested in the women's self-image and she asked them to answer the question 'Who am I?' ten times. One of the women replied as follows:

> "I am a housewife.
> I am going to the shop.
> I am a mother.
> I am a good housewife.
> I am a mother of four children.
> I am a wife.
> I am a good cleaner.
> I am a good washer.
> I am always working."

This woman was a full-time housewife. Do you think women who are mothers today would reply in the same way? (The study was done between 1969 and 1970.) (see Figure 1.12).

As men and women age, gender identity is still important. Women are still seen as more focussed on the family and grandchildren, and may feel that once they are retired they can spend their time with friends and family. They can also be seen as 'natural carers' for family members who are ill or disabled. Men may find it

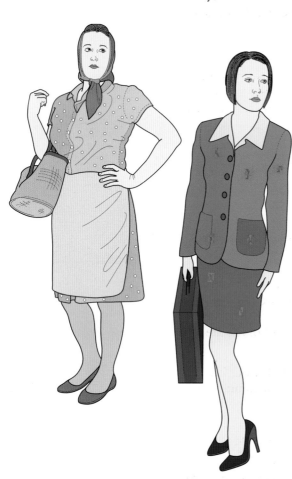

Figure 1.12 Do women today have a different self-image?

> **KEY TERM**
>
> **Gender** – the psychological and social development of male and female roles in a society.

> **KEY TERM**
>
> **Stereotype** – a simplified general image about a particular group of people- 'they all do…'

difficult to adapt to retirement, as they tend to see their work as part of 'who they are'. If they were managers in their workplace, they may try to 'manage' family members, which can lead to problems in the family.

Culture

Culture is related to a system of beliefs, practices, dress, language and religious beliefs, which all influence our self-concept by influencing our feelings of belonging and our ideas about membership of certain social groups. Culture gives us a sense of shared values. Different cultural groups may experience discrimination and this could have an effect on their self-concept.

Emotional Development

Emotional development occurs throughout the life course and is affected by the experiences we have at different times throughout our lives. Emotional development is linked to becoming a confident and stable adult with high self-esteem. Research shows that children who have had a loving and stable relationship with a parent have higher self-esteem than those who have had a poor experience in childhood.

Education

Education can affect your self-concept. If teachers tell you that you are lazy or not very clever, this will have an effect on the way you see yourself and have a negative impact on your self-image and your performance at school. On the other hand, if a teacher praises you and tells you that you will succeed, this will have increase your positive self-image and give you high self-esteem.

Relationships with others

Relationships with other people are very important throughout our lives. Friends and family can make us feel supported and happy about ourselves. However, if relationships break down or we feel people are behaving badly towards us, this can affect our self-image.

Sexual orientation

This is the term used in sociology to describe the focus of an individual's sex drive. Homosexual orientation is attraction towards the same sex, i.e. gay men and lesbian women. Although society appears to be more tolerant nowadays, some people may still fear and dislike homosexuals (this is called homophobia) and this may have a negative effect on someone's self-concept.

Life experience

Life experiences can have a positive or negative effect on our self-concept or our self-esteem. In some of the case studies in this chapter, we can see the importance of life experience (see Case Study 2). Although Mary has many problems to cope with because of her blindness, she appears to have made the best of her life experiences.

We can see that all these nine factors affect our self-concept during our life course: from infancy and childhood; school and college life; as an adult with our own families; and in later adult life

ACTIVITY

Look through the nine factors and decide how important they are at each life stage.

Social development across the life stages

Social development includes the ability to communicate and to make relationships with other people.

Table 1.7 shows how social development is a lifelong process.

Life stage	Development
Infants 0–2 years	
0–4 weeks	Baby can follow a moving person with their eyes during the first month of life
1–2 months	Baby can smile at human faces and recognise their mother
2–3 months	Baby can smile and make a noise when an adult or children are near
4–5 months– 2 years	Knows he only has one mother and can identify known and unknown people. Developing relationships with key family members
Early childhood 3–8 years	
3–4 years	Makes friends with other children; develops play skills; is aware if children are male or female
4–8 years	Can think about the feelings of others. Plays with children of the same sex after the age of 8
Adolescence 9–18 years	Friendship groups are very important. After 12-years-of-age children may take on some work roles in the family such as helping with younger siblings and with domestic chores
Early adulthood 19–45 years	Personal friendships widen through contact at college, in leisure time; these may develop into sexual relationships, as well as temporary or permanent partnerships. Career development and marriage and having children may occur. May have to support older members of the family as well as coping with older children, who leave home, or may still be living at home, which can be stressful
Middle adulthood 46–65	As adults get older their friendship groups may become smaller, as people retire and move away, but some long-lasting friendships will remain. This group is seen as the 'in-between' generation who may have the pressure of looking after elderly parents as well as grandchildren
Later adulthood 66 years+	Many adults in their 60s and 70s lead interesting lives once they have retired, but this depends on the money they have and if they have good health. There may be more opportunities to follow their interests. In later adulthood, family relationships become very important again

Table 1.7 Social development is a lifelong process

As we can see in Table 1.7 the relationships we have during our lives are very important to our development. A recent research study (2008) found that people with 10 friends were happier than those with less than five. During our lifetime our friendships may change but many older people have lifelong friends; sadly, many older people may lose touch with their friends as they move away or die, and because of ill-health and lack of mobility older people may become very isolated.

Socialisation

Socialisation is the process of acquiring the knowledge, values and social skills that enable the individual to become an accepted member of his or her social group or society, and to behave according to the rules, customs, and lifestyles of that society.

Primary socialisation takes place within the family, when a child learns how to fit into the family.

Secondary socialisation is socialisation that continues throughout life, throughout school, college and the workplace, as well as through the media, friendship groups and other influences. For example, women's magazines encourage girls and women to behave in a particular way that reflects how women are seen in current UK society.

In this section we can see that there is a very close interlinking of physical, intellectual, emotional and social development in how we develop as individuals.

Factors affecting human growth and development

There are a number of factors that contribute both positively and negatively to health and well-being. These factors can cause individual differences in patterns of growth and development. The factors may be:

- physical
- social, cultural and emotional
- economic
- environmental
- psychological.

There is a summary of these factors in Figure 1.13.

KEY TERM

Primary socialisation – is the socialisation that takes place within the family as the child learns how to fit into the family.

Secondary socialisation – is socialisation that continues throughout life, through school, college, the workplace, as well as through the media, friendship groups and other influences.

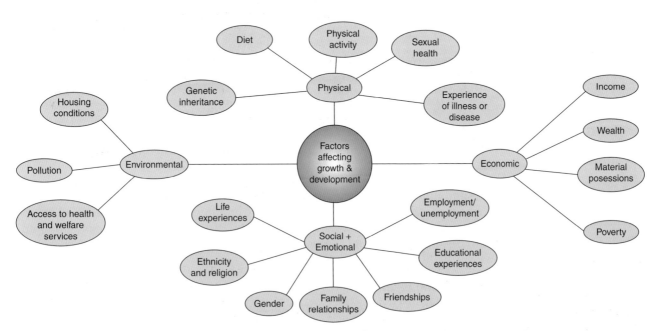

Figure 1.13 Factors that affect growth and development

The different factors may interrelate to cause individual differences in patterns of growth and development.

Physical factors

All human characteristics are determined by either genes, or environmental factors (for example, physical factors, such as diet, or environmental surroundings) or, most commonly, a combination of both genes and environmental factors.

Genetic inheritance

(See also pages 135–36, on 'Genetic inheritance' in Chapter 3).

The genes an individual inherits from their parents will obviously affect their growth and development. Everybody knows, for example, that tall parents are likely to produce tall children and short parents are likely to produce short children. Figure 1.14 shows how a person's height can be predicted from the heights of the parents.

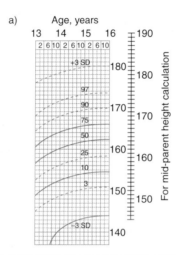
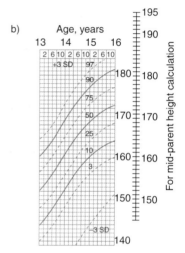

Mid parental centile: To calculate her 'mid-parental' centile, an indicator of her adult stature, mark two heights – her mother's (M) and her father's (F) **MINUS** 12.5 cm (F) – on the vertical line. Read off the height midway between M and F and plot it (X) on the 16-yr line. As an adult, she should be somewhere ±8.5 cm of X.

Mid parental centile: To calculate his 'mid-parental' centile, an indicator of his adult stature, mark two heights – his father's (F) and his mother's **PLUS** 12.5 cm (M) – on the vertical line. Read off the height midway between F and M and plot it (X) on the 16-yr line. As an adult, he should be somewhere ±8.5 cm of X.

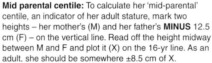

Figure 1.14 Charts to estimate a) girls' and b) boys' adult height from the height of the parents

Some characteristics, such as eye colour, are determined just from the genes a child inherits from their parents, but there is disagreement on the extent to which characteristics such as intelligence and personality are determined by genes and how much they are influenced by the environment a person grows up in. (See 'How genetic and environmental factors can affect growth and development' on page 39, below.)

Illness and disease

Serious illness or disease can affect all aspects of growth and development, for example:

- If the immune system is working to overcome an infectious disease, it uses protein from the diet to make white blood cells and antibodies. This means less protein is available for growth, so growth rate may slow.
- As well as having physical effects, poor health can limit a young person's education, or an older person's employment prospects.

- Studies have shown that children with chronic (long term) disease are likely to be less socially outgoing than healthy children, and have more problems relating to their peers.
- People with chronic illness are more likely to suffer from depression than the general population.

(See also pages 135–36, on '*Genetic inheritance*' in Chapter 3 which includes information on genetic diseases.)

Diet

(See also the section on '*Diet*', Chapter 3, page 137, that explains the positive and negative influences of nutrition on health and well-being.) Table 1.8 shows what we need in our diet for healthy growth and development, and what we should avoid.

You need		Avoid	
Energy (Carbohydrates and fats)	Amount will depend on level of activity; age; size; gender; pregnancy or breast feeding	Too much energy (fats and carbohydrates)	Causes obesity
Protein	For growth, repair and a healthy immune system	Too much saturated fat	Causes heart disease
Vitamins and minerals	For healthy growth and development (see Chapter 3, pages 137–40)	Too much salt	Causes high blood pressure
Fibre	Keeps food moving through the gut	Some food additives (see article below)	Causes hyperactivity and impair learning
Water	Prevents dehydration		

Table 1.8 Diet and development

Height and diet

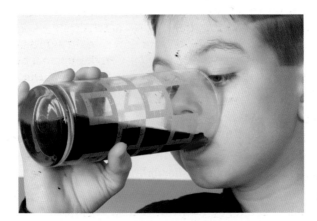

Figure 1.15 Artificial food colourings are thought to cause hyperactivity in some children

Average height in the UK increased in the last century; for example, in 1750 the average young male height was about 160 cm, and in 2006 it was 176.7 cm (163.7 cm for females). It is thought that improved diet, particularly an increase in protein, is the main reason for this increase in height. Poor nutrition is common in areas of poverty, and it can be seen that in poorer countries the average adult height is less than that in richer countries.

Food additives and intellectual development

As the article (Guardian 9/4/08) below shows, there is concern that the use of some artificial colourings causes hyperactive behaviour in children (see Figure 1.15). Children showing hyperactive behaviour find it difficult to sit still and concentrate, so they cannot learn effectively.

ACTIVITY

Use www.action on additives.com/Food_additives/More_information/ to find out which foods the six artificial additives mentioned in the article are found in.

'Food watchdog seeks ban on six artificial colourings'

Companies asked to eliminate use before 2010

Research highlights links to hyperactive behaviour

'The Food Standards Agency wants six artificial colourings to be removed from food and drink made in Britain. . . because of 'an accumulating body of evidence' suggesting that their use is associated with hyperactive behaviour in children.*

The Food and Drink Federation, an industry trade body, confirmed the industry had been working on removing colourings 'for a number of years' but said there were still technical difficulties finding alternative ingredients for some products.

The colourings involved are sunset yellow (E110), quinoline yellow (E104), carmoisine (E122), allura red (E129), tatrazine (E102) and ponceau (E124).

Hyperactivity is a behaviour officially indicated by increased movement, impulsiveness and inattention, and can impair learning.'

Source: Guardian 9/4/08

Exercise

(See also the section *'Exercise'* in Chapter 3, pages 140–1 that explains the influence of physical activity and lack of physical activity on health and well-being.)

Exercise is essential for healthy growth and development for a number of reasons:

- it strengthens muscles, bones and joints
- it improves balance, coordination, flexibility and posture
- it prevents obesity
- it reduces the chance of heart disease in later life
- it develops self-esteem by creating a strong sense of purpose and self-fulfillment
- team sports teach how to interact and cooperate with others.

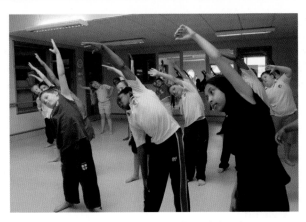

Figure 1.16 Exercise is essential for healthy growth and development

Alcohol

(See also the section *'Alcohol'* in Chapter 3, pages 142–5 that explains its influence on health and well-being.)

Alcohol can affect growth and development throughout the lifespan.

There is generally agreement that women should avoid alcohol in pregnancy, as it affects the growth and development of the foetus. If the mother drinks excessively, the baby may be born with foetal alcohol syndrome (FAS). Symptoms include:

- small eyes
- increased risk of cleft palate
- 'pug' nose
- severe learning difficulties
- problems with sight and hearing
- smaller-than-average birth weight
- problems with growth and development
- increased risk of long-term health problems.

There is increasing evidence that repeated exposure to alcohol during adolescence (binge drinking) can lead to long-lasting effects on cognitive abilities, including learning, memory and attention span. Research suggests that alcohol use by teenagers can affect brain development and that the effects could be permanent. ('How Binge Drinking Affects the Teenage Brain', *Alcohol Anonymous Reviews*, 4 Feb 2009)

Smoking

(See the section *'Smoking'* in Chapter 3, pages 145–7) that explains its influence on health and well-being.)

Like alcohol, smoking can affect growth and development throughout the lifespan.

If a mother smokes, her baby will have a lower-than-average birth weight and will be more likely to be placed in intensive care when it is born. If a baby has a low birth weight, this may have a long-term affect on the child's growth and development.

It is widely known that 'smoking stunts your growth', but now there is good evidence that it also affects brain development and therefore intellectual ability. In 1947 around 465 people had their mental abilities assessed when they were aged 11. When they reached age 64 they were assessed again. It was found that the smokers performed less well than the non-smokers, even when other factors such as education and alcohol consumption were taken into consideration.

Social, cultural and emotional factors

Social factors

We have already seen that our emotional and social development is affected by the relationships we have, as well as our biological and genetic make up.

Social factors include the following:

- the family we are born into
- the friends we have from early school days to later life
- the type of school we go to
- the educational opportunities we have
- the qualifications we achieve
- the type of work we do
- the type of community we live in – urban or rural
- the religion we may belong to, or the belief system we have
- whether we are male or female
- what ethnic group we belong to
- our sexual orientation.

All these factors may be related to economic influences.

KEY TERM

Ascribed class – this is the class you are born into and your ascribed social class will affect whatever you do in life – the school you go to, the friends you have, the lifestyle and the job you have.

Family

The family we are born into will determine what happens to us during the rest of our lives. Although we are supposed to live in a classless society, most people remain in the social class they have been born into. (See 'Occupation and social class' in Chapter 3 page 155.)

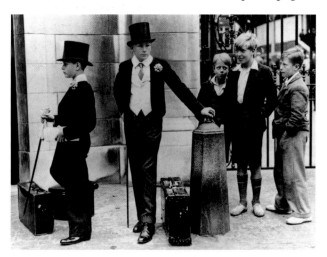

Figure 1.17 Class divisions still occur

Unless offered a scholarship, only rich people can afford to go to a public school like Eton (see Figure 1.17). If you want to learn a musical instrument, this has economic costs in the purchase of instruments and having lessons – not everyone can afford this. Your family may not be able to support you in college or university. Studies have shown that the qualifications you have are important in determining what job you may do, but your ascribed class status is even more important, as the social networks set up through your family and your education can support you throughout your life.

Studies among doctors show that many doctors are the sons of doctors, and this is the same in other professions. If your father has a working class job, you may be more likely to be in a similar job.

Class divisions are changing, as the number of traditional working class jobs in factories, farms and fishing have reduced a great deal, so that young people may end up in more middle class positions because there aren't the working class jobs available.

We can see from these examples that social factors are very closely linked to economic factors, but they can also be linked to lifestyle factors which may affect health and well-being.

Friends

The section on 'Friendships' on page 43, below, explains that friendships are important social relationships. Friends can provide important emotional support and are very important for our emotional and social health and well-being.

Educational experiences

(See also the section in Chapter 3 on *'Educational experiences,'* page 149) which explains the importance of education in health and well-being.)

A poor education is likely to affect a person's life opportunities. Research shows that there are not equal educational opportunities for children, for example:

- Children who are from poorer families are less likely to achieve good qualifications
  - Young people from poorer areas of the country are much more likely to leave school with fewer qualifications and much less likely to go onto higher education.
  - Pupils who are eligible for free school meals perform less well in each Key Stage and at GCSE than pupils who are not eligible for free school meals; for example, in 2007 the figures of those achieving 5+ GCSE grades A*–C were 35.5% (free school meals) compared with 62.8% (not eligible for free school meals).

- There is variation in the educational achievements of different ethnic groups

- Children in care have a lower level of achievement than others
  - Almost a third of children in care take no GCSEs, compared with 1% of all children
  - Only 13% of these children obtained five good GCSEs, compared with 62% of all children
  - 28% of these children had statements of special educational need, compared with 3% of children generally.

People with poor qualifications are likely to suffer greater job insecurity, poorer working conditions and to suffer more unemployment and receive a lower income. Although there are exceptions, for most people their schooling affects their future economic status and income.

> **KEY TERM**
>
> Children in care – Children looked after by social services either in their own homes, by foster parents, or in residential care.

Employment/unemployment

(See also the section on *'Employment status'*, on page 32, below, and the sections in Chapter 3 on *'Employment/unemployment'* and *'Employment status'*.)

Employment can benefit a person in a number of ways, other than providing an income. For example:

- some types of employment which involve physical activity may contribute to physical fitness
- a person may feel intellectually stimulated by their employment
- it is likely that employment will provide opportunities for socialising and friendship.

Community involvement

Some commentators on the way people work and live in communities stress the importance of a sense of community that has shared values and supports the people living within it. This view is supported by a German philosopher called Tonnies (1855–1936), who put forward the view that people in small communities like villages and small towns, develop good relationships with each other and this is of benefit to everyone in the community. But he felt that large towns and cities could not develop this sense of community. People in large cities could find it difficult to develop close personal relationships and this could have a negative effect on people.

Community involvement can be seen to have a positive effect on personal development. Activity within the community can be for all ages and areas. Local councils are now recognising that it is important to involve local people in making decisions about a range of plans – such as plans for sheltered housing, schools that are being built, as well as the development of shopping centres, and other facilities used by the residents. Some districts have organised local committee meetings when council officers meet with residents to discuss proposed changes. In one London borough the parks department consulted the local people about developing a skateboarding park. The young people who would use the park gave their opinion about how the skate park should be organised, and they are on a committee to review the building and use of the park. Examples of community involvement can include involving groups that are 'hard to reach'. In one area a large centre was opened that was to be used by different groups – so one day the local Euro–Asian group took over the café and provided food for anyone who wanted to come; in the evening the hall was used by young people learning kung fu. In the same building, a dementia café takes place at weekends when dementia patients and their carers can come and relax and have lunch, while volunteers help with the patients so that the carers have a rest.

KEY TERM

Culture – Culture relates to the way of life of a particular society or group. It can include the following aspects:

- the language used – both spoken and written
- the customs followed – lifestyle and religion
- a shared system of values – beliefs and morals
- social norms – acceptable patterns of behaviour, including dress and diet.

Cultural factors

Cultural factors may affect every aspect of your life. Culture can be about a whole society or a part of society.

Look at the leisure activities listed below. Who do you think are more likely to attend these? Think about the social class divisions we have already discussed when you are thinking about the answers

- go to the Henley regatta
- go greyhound racing
- go on holiday to Scotland
- go on holiday to Spain using a cheap flight offer
- go to the opera
- go to an Elvis impressionist show
- have fish and chips and a beer
- have Lobster Thermidor in an expensive restaurant.

We could say these divisions are using stereotypes but you can see how cultural differences can dictate how we live our lives. There are also stereotypes of what a middle class family is and what a working class family is.

Do you remember the key term stereotype?

Religion

Religion can be defined as a system of belief that influences the way we think and act; if we have religious beliefs we may go to church, or mosque or to other group events where we take part in collective worship.

Religion can be seen as an important influence in a society. This influence can be positive. It can make someone feel supported and helped by being part of a group. However, religion can also cause problems when conflict may occur between different religious groups.

CASE STUDY 1 – Ann

Ann came to London to do her nursing training. Ann had no family and had been in care since she was 4-years-old. When she came to London she felt very lonely. One of the girls in her group invited her to go to a party that was being held at the local Baptist church. Ann was welcomed by the people there and she felt part of a 'family' in the church, so she went regularly after that. If anyone asked her why she went to church she always said, 'I feel I belong to a family now, by belonging to the church'.

The numbers of people attending church in the UK has fallen. Religion has become more of a personal matter. The UK is seen as a Christian country and the Queen is Head of the Church of England. However, nowadays there is a range of different religions. You may have studied these at school. People who have a strong religious belief may find that they can cope better with problems in their lives. Most religions mark events in life with particular rituals. Birth, puberty, marriage and death are key times. In the Christian religion these events would include christening the child and confirmation of the teenager. Marriage and death would be marked by church services. Members of the Jewish faith mark puberty with special ceremonies for boys (bar mitzvah) (see Figure 1.18). These rituals give those people taking part a way of expressing their support to the person who is going through these ceremonies.

Marriage rituals confirm the couple's attachment to each other and by taking vows at the service this shows their intention to take married life seriously. Many people find they feel more secure in a marriage. Recent reports show that marriages last longer than relationships in which couples cohabit. There are various rituals carried out when someone is dying, such as prayers and anointing the person with oil. This can give comfort to the relatives, as well as a feeling of acceptance for the dying person.

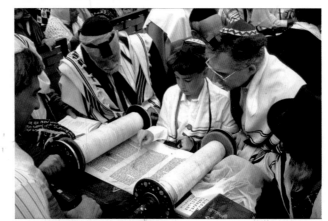

Figure 1.18 Boy at his bar mitzvah

Gender

We have already seen how gender affects our self-concept (see pages 18–19). Gender still remains a key aspect of our development. The roles of men and women have changed since the 1950s, due to women having access to education and jobs that were previously thought to be for men only. However, the roles of men and women in marriage and in other relationships are still very much determined by gender. One thing that can never change is that at the moment only women can have babies and this has an impact on their development and relationships throughout their lives.

Ethnicity

It is important for health and social care workers to be aware of cultural differences between different ethnic groups. These differences need to be considered when looking after patients, as they will influence the roles of a couple in marriage, the diet and dress seen as acceptable and rituals about aspects of care such as birth, circumcision, becoming an adult and dying. If you are born into a particular ethnic group, this will have a major impact on your personal development and your life chances.

Sexual orientation

Sexual orientation is a further aspect of personal development that is seen to be relevant in the UK today.

Heterosexual orientation is when a person is attracted to the opposite sex. Homosexual orientation is attraction towards the same sex – gay men and lesbian women. Homosexual activity was seen to be illegal in the UK until The Sexual Offences Act of 1967 when homosexual acts between men over the age of 21 was allowed. In 1993 the House of Commons voted to lower the age of consent for homosexual men from 21 to 18. In 2000 it was lowered to 16.

In the discussion on gender, girls and boys are supposed to behave in certain ways, with the emphasis on heterosexual behaviour, and this emphasis can cause problems for homosexuals; they may be picked on at work and in everyday life, and be the subject of bullying. This can affect one's self-concept and personal development.

Relationship formation

Later on this chapter, we will look at factors such as marriage and divorce (see pages 41–42) and how these aspects affect personal development.

Emotional factors

As we have already seen on page 15–16 emotional development takes place throughout life, and happy stable relationships encourage healthy personal development.

Economic factors

(See also the section in Chapter 3 on 'Economic factors', page 154–5, that explain the importance of income, wealth, material possessions, employment status, occupation and social class on health, well-being and life opportunities.)

Economic factors affect growth and development because people need resources (money, income, wealth) to pay for things that are essential, such as food,

---

KEY TERM

Sexual orientation – a term used in sociology to describe the focus of an individual's sex drive.

clothing and housing. People may also want further resources for items that they desire but are not essential, such as designer-label clothing, meals in restaurants or expensive holidays. The ways in which people are able to obtain and use their money will have a significant effect on their health, welfare and self-concept.

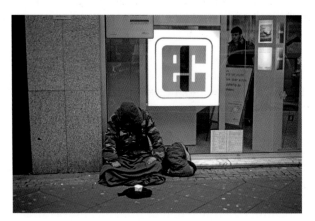

Figure 1.19 Economic factors affect health and development

Income and wealth

(See also 'Material possessions' including 'Wants and needs' Activity on page 35–7.)

Income

The main income for many people is their wage from employment, but other sources of income include benefits, pensions, rents, interest from savings and dividends from shares. The higher an individual's or household's income, the less likely they are to live in poverty, so the healthier they are likely to be (see pages 35 and 154–5 to find out why poverty can be so detrimental to health and well-being). It is also likely that the higher an individual's or household's income, the more material possessions they will have, and the effect of that is also described below. A Scottish study published in 2007 showed that households with low annual incomes are more than three time more likely to have someone with a long-term illness, health problem or disability than a high income household.

In times of recession, there is evidence that life expectancy falls and rates of mental illness increase. This seems to particularly affect men who suffer a drop in income because:

- if they believe in traditional gender roles, in which the man is seen as the provider, they may feel a loss of identity;
- they are less likely to talk about their feelings, which can increase the risk of depression or even suicide.

Most people would agree that some variation in income is fair as it reflects differences in factors such as skill, training, responsibility and risk. However, excessive differences lead to social inequalities. Recently, there has been criticism of the size of the bonuses paid to some people working in the city and of the salaries of some CEOs (Chief Executive Officers) compared with those of their staff.

> **KEY TERM**
>
> **Income** – the sum of all earnings of a household or individual in a given period of time.
>
> **Wealth** – the extent of an individual's or household's possessions and resources.

In 2008 the Joseph Rowntree Foundation, a social policy research and development charity, estimated that a single person living in Britain would need to earn at least £13, 400 a year before tax for a minimum standard of living. A couple with two children would need £370 a week and a pensioner couple would need £201 excluding housing and childcare costs. The Foundation's definition of a minimum standard of living was not just what money would be needed for survival (food, clothes and shelter), but also what was needed to buy items to give people the 'opportunities and choices to participate in society'. Examples of these items include:

- For a single person – walking boots, a 'pay-as-you-go' mobile and a bicycle
- For a pensioner couple – an occasional meal in a restaurant and a bird-feeder
- For a single mother – nappies and a Christmas tree
- For families – a one-week self-catering holiday in the UK and a home computer

A car or cigarettes were considered not to be essential items.

Wealth

Wealth means something slightly different from income because it refers to the total value of the possessions held by an individual (or society). Some possessions, such as a small business, factory or farm, can be a source of income for the people they belong to.

Wealth can be considered as a way in which inequalities in society are passed from one generation to the next. In America, for example, over half the wealthiest people have inherited family fortunes. If students have their university education paid for by parents or grandparents, or if a young person is given financial help from relatives to buy a house, they are benefiting from wealth accumulated by previous generations and have an advantage over those from less wealthy families. Wealth can give an individual more choices and greater power.

There is a relationship between wealth and class (See 'Social class and occupation, pages 33–4).

- Upper class: most people from this class will have inherited their wealth, and wealth will be more important than income.
- Middle class: most people from this class will be more likely to rely on income than accumulated wealth.
- Working class: most people from this class will have a limited income and few opportunities to accumulate any wealth.

There are people who think that in addition to possessions, we should also include health and spiritual well-being when considering how wealthy a person is.

Employment status

The sections in Chapter 3 on 'Employment/Unemployment' (pages 150–1) and 'Employment status' (page 155) and 'Employment/unemployment' in this chapter (on pages 54–6), explain the importance of employment in health, well-being and life opportunities. Employment does not just help a person to be financially better off; it can provide supportive relationships, self-esteem and education. There is evidence that those in employment have better physical and mental health than those who are unemployed.

Social class and occupation

Social class is used to indicate the economic and social circumstances of an individual. It is made up of a number of related elements including:

- economic characteristics, such as wealth, income and occupation
- political characteristics, such as social status and power
- cultural characteristics such as lifestyle, values, beliefs and level of education.

There are different ways of defining which social class an individual belongs to, but usually it is measured in terms of occupation. In 2000 the Standard Occupational Classification (SOC2000) was produced. However, this has 353 groups, so a simpler version has been produced by the Office for National Statistics that only has five classes (see Table 1.9 below).

Class	Label	Examples
1	Managerial and professional occupations	Company directors, Doctors, Solicitors, Librarians, Police, Social workers, Teachers, Nurses and midwives, Journalists, Actors
2	Intermediate occupations	Secretaries, Driving instructors, Computer operators, Telephone fitters
3	Small employers and own account workers	Publicans, Play group leaders, Farmers, Taxi drivers, Window cleaners
4	Lower supervisory and technical occupations	Printers, Plumbers, Butchers, Bus inspectors, Train drivers
5	Semi-routine and routine occupations	Shop assistants, Traffic wardens, Cooks, Hairdressers, Postal workers, Waiters, Road sweepers, Cleaners, Building labourers, Refuse collectors

Table 1.9 The five-class version of the National Statistics Socio-economic Classification (NS-SEC)

- No account is taken of relative earnings.
- Occupations have been sorted on the basis of factors such as job security and promotion opportunities.
- There is also a category for those who have never had any employment and the long-term unemployed.

The social class to which we belong may have implications for our growth and development. This is mainly because of the link between social class and poverty.

People in lower social classes, including children, are more likely to suffer from:

- infective and parasitic diseases
- pneumonia
- poisonings
- violence.

Adults in lower social classes are more likely to suffer from:

- cancer
- heart disease

- respiratory disease
- depression and other mental health problems.

The reasons for the health inequalities between the different social classes can be complex, but the factors given in the list below are likely to have an effect:

● Poverty (see below on page 35)	It is likely that people in lower social classes will have less regular employment and a lower income than those in higher social classes. It is likely that people in poverty will have poorer diets and housing, both of which lead to poorer health.
● Poor access to the knowledge and resources that maintain health	Health promotion messages are less likely to reach people in the lower social classes. They are also likely to have a lower NHS allocation.
● Poor working conditions	Manual workers have a higher level of diseases associated with hazards such as chemicals, dust and noise. They are also more likely to suffer accidents a work and to suffer stress brought on by carrying out boring, repetitive tasks.
● Smoking	The lower a person's social class, the more likely they are to smoke (see Figure 1.20). For example, manual workers are more than twice as likely to smoke as those from the professional classes. Suggested reasons for this are: ● People from lower social classes are influenced less by health promotion messages. ● People from lower social classes are likely to suffer more stress which they attempt to counteract by smoking. Figure 1.20 There is a correlation between social class and smoking

ACTIVITY

1. Do you consider that you belong to a particular social class? If so, which one? What are your reasons for your decision?
2. Two suggestions are given for the higher likelihood of smoking amongst people from lower social classes compared with higher social classes. Do you agree with these, and can you suggest others?
3. Recently the Prime Minister said, 'A child's social class background at birth is still the best predictor of how well he or she will do at school and later on in life'.

Discuss what is being done, or could be done, to improve the achievement of children from lower social classes at school and later in life.

Poverty

Poverty is a state in which, for an individual or family, there is either a lack of resources sufficient to maintain a healthy existence (absolute poverty) or a lack of resources sufficient to achieve a standard of living considered acceptable in that particular society (relative poverty). In 2006–7, 2.5 million pensioners and 2.9 million children were living in poverty in the UK.

Children born in the poorest parts of Britain die, on average, many years before children from wealthier areas. For example:

- A boy born in the Carlton district of Glasgow is likely to die 28 years earlier than one born a few miles away in Lenzie.
- Boys born in the wealthy London suburb of Hampstead are likely to live 11 years longer than children born in Kings Cross.

Table 1.10 shows some of the inequalities that children from poorer families face.

	Richest 20%	Poorest 20%
Have a safe outdoor play space	96%	74%
Go swimming at least once a month	73%	47%
Have friends round for tea every month	81%	63%
One week's family holiday a year	94%	40%
Go to play group once a week	86%	51%

Table 1.10 Children's access to facilities based on family income

(Source: The Guardian 11/6/08)

ACTIVITY

Find out about the government's pledge to eradicate child poverty by 2020 and the work of the Campaign to End Child Poverty, a coalition of 120 organisations.

Material possessions

Material possessions are the things someone owns. Some material possessions are obviously necessary to survive, and material possessions, for example, a car, may make it easier for people to control their lives and participate more fully in society. more. However, some people argue that:

- more material possessions do not necessarily make a person happier
- some material possessions act as 'status symbols' that people may be judged on
- many material possessions have an adverse effect on the environment
- advertisers and manufacturers ensure that people are never satisfied for long with their belongings.

Psychologists say that the pleasure from a new purchase fades within two to three months. People may then buy more things to renew the positive feelings from their material possessions. This can create a 'vicious circle' in which a person feels unhappy and insecure and constantly spends more than they can really afford.

KEY TERM

Material possessions – the things a person owns

Consumerism – equating personal happiness with material possessions

Research has shown that experiences such as holidays make people happier than possessions; are more likely to lead to social interaction; and lead to a greater sense of vitality, both at the time and when remembering the experience.

ACTIVITY

The amount of money, income or material possessions needed for a healthy and happy life varies from person to person.

Game – wants or needs?

Step One

Look at Table 1.11. You will see that there are a number of suggestions for the economic resources we may want or need to live healthily and happily in this society. Make a photocopy of the table for each small group playing the game, and cut out the 28 suggestion boxes.

Step Two

After discussion, each group should then place each suggestion into one of two piles labelled as follows:

1. Economic resources we **need** to live healthily and happily.
2. Economic resources we may **want** to live healthily and happily.

No suggestion should be placed in either category unless all group members agree. Where there is a difference in opinion, the members of the group must justify their choice and attempt to persuade the others that their choice is the right one. If no agreement can be reached, the reasons should be recorded by the group and that suggestion omitted from the final piles.

Step Three

Each group tells the others which suggestions they have placed in their lists and differences can be noted and discussed. The whole class can decide on where any omitted suggestions from each group should go.

Step Four

Follow up this game by researching the following questions:

1. In the UK, what is the average annual salary, before tax (see www.statistics.gov.uk)? How much is this per week?

2. What income from benefits could an unemployed man or woman in their twenties expect to receive per week in the UK today (see www.direct.gov.uk)?

3. What does the current state pension pay per week to:
   - a single man or woman?
   - a married couple?

4. Go to www.jrf.org.uk, the website of The Joseph Rowntree Foundation, the well-respected social policy research and development charity mentioned in the section on 'Income', above. Use this website to find further details of what items the Foundation considers necessary for a minimum standard of living and what levels of income would be needed to provide these.

A	B	C	D
1 Enough income to buy (and replace when worn out/outgrown) a set of basic clothing from second-hand/charity shops or similar, e.g. jumble sales: Approx. £200.00 per person per year.	**1** Enough income to make (sew. knit etc.) most of your own clothes and to buy the rest. Approx. £300.00 per person per year.	**1** Enough income to buy (and replace when worn out/outgrown) a set of new basic clothing from high street stores or equivalent, e.g. mail order. Approx £600.00 per person per year.	**1** Enough income to buy (and replace when worn out/outgrown) a set of clothing from designer shops/with designer lables. Approx £1200.00 per person per year.
2 Enough income to afford a weekly food/household goods bills of £20.00–£30.00 per person.	**2** Enough income to afford a weekly food/household goods bill of £30.00–£40.00 per person.	**2** Enough income to afford a weekly food/household goods bill of £40.00–£50.00 per person.	**2** Enough income to afford to spend as much as you like on food and household goods plus resturant and Lake-away bills.
3 Enough income to afford to buy, after all other essentials have been paid for, up to 4 second-class postage stamps a week. Approx. £1.00–£2.00 per person.	**3** Enough income to afford to buy, after all other essentials have been paid for, birthday/Christmas/ other religious festival presents for close family. Approx. £80.00 per person per year.	**3** Enough income to afford to buy, after all other essentials have been paid for, up to ten units of alcohol a week and/or twenty cigarettes a day. Approx. £35.00–50.00 per person per week.	**3** Enough income to afford to buy personal private health insurance. Between £500.00–1000.00 per person per year.
4 Enough income to buy, insure and maintain a second hand pedal bicycle with safety helmet and puncture kit. Approx. £150.00 per person in the year the bicycle is bought.	**4** Enough annual income to afford to pay off a monthly loan on, tax, insure, service and buy petrol for a small second-hand car. Approx. £1800.00 per person in the year the car is bought.	**4** Enough annual income to afford to pay off a monthly loan on, tax, insure, service and buy petrol for a small new car. Approx. £4000.00 per person in the year the car is bought.	**4** Enough income to afford to buy outright, tax, insure, service and run a new car. Anything above £12,000.00 in the year the car is bought.
5 Enough income to rent a room in a hostel or night shelter.	**5** Enough income to rent a flat/house from a council, a housing association, private landlord or a co-operative.	**5** Enough income to borrow money from a building society, bank or other lender (this is called a mortgage) to buy a house or flat. You will usually be allowed to borrow two and a half to three times your annual gross income, i.e. before tax.	**5** Enough income to buy your house outright.
6 Enough income to afford a weekly T.V. rental payment and annual T.V. license bill. Approx. £200.00 a year per person.	**6** Enough income to afford to buy a new T.V. and video and pay the annual T.V license fee. Approx. £300.00–400.00 per person in the year the T.V. and video were bought.	**6** Enough income to buy a home computer and software and pay for fax, e-mail and Internet services plus subscriptions to satellites, cable and digital T.V. Approx. £1500.00–2000.00 in the year the computer was bought.	**6** Enough income to afford to buy outright any combination of T.V., video, computer, fax, games console, software, printers etc. the individual or family desires. Approx. £5000.00+ in the year the items are bought.
7 Employment pay and/ or social security benefit/ pension which gives an income (after tax) of £80.00 plus housing benefit per person per week.	**7** Employment pay and/ or social security benefit/ pension which gives an income (after tax) of £130.00–250.00 a week.	**7** Employment pay and/ or social security benefit/ pension which gives an income (after tax) of £400.00–500.00 per person per week.	**7** Income and earning which give a weekly income (after tax) of more than £600.00 per person per week.

Table 1.11 Suggestion boxes – wants or needs?

Physical environment factors

Pollution

The section in Chapter 3 on *'Pollution'* (pages 156-8) explains the detrimental effect that pollution can have on health and well-being.

Noise

The section in Chapter 3 on *'Noise'* (page 158) explains the detrimental effect that noise can have on health and well-being.

Housing conditions

The section in Chapter 3 on *'Housing'* (pages 158–160) explains the important influence of housing conditions on health and well-being.

Rural/urban lifestyle

The section in Chapter 3 on *'Rural/urban lifestyle'* (pages 161–3) explains the effect that a rural or urban lifestyle can have on health and well-being.

Psychological factors

Psychological factors are to do with the feelings people have about themselves and others and the events that happen to them.

Stress

The section in Chapter 3 on *'Stress'* (pages 163–5) explains the effect of both short- and long-term stress on health and well-being. A constant high level of stress will lead to physical, emotional and intellectual ill-health, so growth and development will be adversely affected.

Treatment may include mild anti-depressants but usually relaxation techniques can help. (See pages 164–5, Chapter 3.)

Relationships with family, friends and partners

You can see in the section, *'The Effects of relationships on personal growth and development'* (see pages 39–47) that relationships are an important aspect of our lives. They offer practical and emotional support, and make us feel happy about ourselves.

Relationships change as we get older and our lives change. Change and development can be positive, but it can also be difficult to cope with if we do not have support. If relationships break down, people can feel sad, lonely, angry and negative about themselves. This can lead to behaviour such as drinking too much, smoking and using drugs, over- or under-eating. People can feel isolated and withdraw from social contact with others. If you feel isolated and upset, this can have an effect on your ability to concentrate on your work or study. People may become depressed and develop physical symptoms such as headaches, tiredness and difficulty in sleeping.

It would seem that supportive relationships with family and friends are very important for our general well-being and that when these relationships break down the effects can be very negative.

How these factors affect self-concept

We have seen the factors that affect a person's self concept (see pages 16–19). We need to concentrate on how we can develop our own self-esteem and see ourselves in a good light. Sometimes it is best to avoid situations (and perhaps certain people!) that reduce our sense of self-worth. Although we may not be able to change certain social factors, such as our age, gender or ethnicity, we may be able to change the way we react to situations and seek support from friends and family to feel valued by others.

How genetic and environmental factors can affect growth and development

- Some characteristics, such as eye colour or diseases, such as cystic fibrosis, are determined entirely by genes.
- A few factors are determined entirely by environment; for example, hair length will depend on how it is cut.
- As mentioned in the section '*Genetic inheritance*', on page 22, above, most aspects of growth and development are influenced by both genes and the environment. The genes a person inherits from their parents will give them the potential to develop certain characteristics; for example, a certain height, or a condition such as coronary heart disease. Their environment will then influence the development of the characteristic; for example diet will influence the actual height an individual grows to, and factors such as diet, smoking and stress will affect whether a person actually suffers from heart disease.

ACTIVITY

i) Sort the following list of characteristics into those determined entirely by genes, those controlled entirely by environment, and those determined partly by genes and partly by the environment:
- Weight
- Intelligence
- Foot size
- Blood group
- Sex (male or female)
- Skin colour
- Breast cancer
- Language spoken.

ii) It is agreed that both genes and environment influence intelligence. Discuss what environmental factors may influence intelligence.

The effects of relationships on personal growth and development

Throughout our lives, from birth until death, we are in different types of relationships.

Key relationships that occur during our lives include the following:

- family relationships – such as marriage, divorce, parenthood, sibling relationships and blended families
- friendships
- intimate personal and sexual relationships
- working relationships.

Family relationships

The family can be defined as 'a social group linked by ties of blood and marriage'. The nuclear family consists of one man, one woman and their dependent children (see Figure 1.21), but nowadays family forms vary considerably.

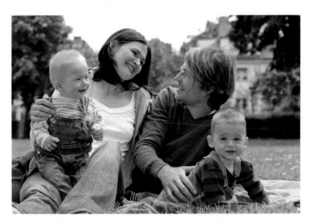

Figure 1.21 The nuclear family

Head of Households in Great Britain	Year (numbers %)				
	1971 (in %)	1981 (in %)	1991 (in %)	2001 (in %)	2007[1] (in %)
One Person					
Under state pension age[1]	6	8	11	14	14
Over state pension age	12	14	16	15	15
One family households					
Couple[2]					
No children	27	26	28	29	28
1–2 dependent children[3]	26	25	20	19	18
3 or more dependent children[3]	9	6	5	4	3
Non-dependent children only	8	8	8	6	7
Lone parent[2]					
Dependent children[3]	3	5	6	7	7
Non-dependent children only	4	4	4	3	3
Two or more unrelated adults	4	5	3	3	3
Multi-family households	1	1	1	1	1
All households					
(=100%) (millions)	18.6	20.2	22.4	23.8	24.4

1 State pension age is currently 65 for men and 60 for women.
2 Other individuals who were not family members may also be included.
3 May also include non-dependent children.

Source: *Census, Labour Force Survey, Office for National Statistics*

Table 1.12 The types of family forms in Great Britain between 1971 and 2007

ACTIVITY

Look at Table 1.12 and describe what you see.

We can see that the number of single parents has increased and the numbers of people living on their own has also increased.

The family has been traditionally seen as providing the following functions:

- teaching children values, attitudes and rules of social behaviour
- supporting the emotional development of the child from infancy to adulthood
- offering stability and security (this could include economic support)
- protecting the health and well-being of all its members.

Family relationships are said to be primary relationships because the people in the family know each other very well, they relate to each other on an informal basis, and one person in the relationship cannot be replaced.

Family relationships are affected by death, divorce and the separation of parents. Since 1990–91 there has been an increase in cohabitation among all age groups. Men are more likely than women to be single, but less likely to be divorced, separated or widowed. This reflects the evidence that men are more likely than women to remarry after losing a partner through death or divorce, and women are more likely to outlive their husbands.

Great Britain	Year (Numbers in %)				
	1972	1981	1997	2001	2007
Couple families					
1 child	16	18	17	17	18
2 children	35	41	37	37	36
3 or more children	41	29	25	24	22
Lone mother families					
1 child	2	3	6	6	7
2 children	2	4	7	8	8
3 or more children	2	3	6	6	6
Lone father families					
1 child	1	1	1	1	
2 or more children	1	1	1	1	1
All children[3]	100	100	100	100	100

Source: *Census, General Household Survey, Labour Force Survey, Office for National Statistics*

Table 1.13 Dependent children by family type

Table 1.13 shows the percentage of children living in different family forms. We can see that the traditional couple family is still the most common type of family in which dependent children live.

At different stages of our lives certain events can have a significant effect on our personal growth and development.

ACTIVITY

Describe the patterns you see.

Marriage

This is a key event; when a couple marries they become a family unit and leave their birth family in order to set up on their own. Although this can be a very happy event, there can be difficulties in becoming accepted by the 'in laws'. There are a lot of 'mother in law' jokes about the older women interfering with the way the new couples start married life

Divorce

Divorce rates have increased since the Divorce Reform Act of 1969 when divorce became easier to arrange. The rise of divorce could be said to show that the family is under threat. A range of changes, such as reliable birth control methods, women going to university and having careers, expectations of women themselves to be economically independent, and the development of welfare payments for divorced or single parents, has meant that women can be independent. In spite of all these changes in attitudes towards women and divorce, many people find that divorce has a negative impact on their personal development. Divorce rates among older couples who have been married for over 20 years have increased. Older women who have spent years of their lives looking after the family may feel that they have nothing to look forward to once the children have left home. They may find it difficult to find work. The division of the home and possessions of the couple may be very difficult.

Parenthood

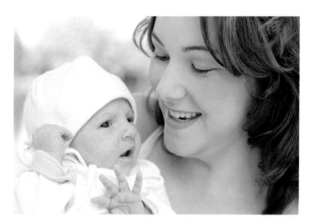

Figure 1.22 The first child

The transition from being a couple who can go out together and have a social life, holidays and be alone together, to being parents who are responsible for a child 24 hours a day, 7 days a week can be difficult. If the birth is difficult, if there is little social or emotional support so that the new parents can have time to go out together and have a break, or if there are financial difficulties, this can put pressure on the marriage. Nowadays, women are encouraged to go back to work after having a baby, so the mother could feel she is doing a 'double shift' of earning money and also caring for the baby. She may feel torn between looking after her child full time or going back to work, so this can be very stressful.

Sibling Relationships

Sibling rivalry – research has shown that the first-born child often feels jealousy towards younger brothers and sisters in the baby's first year, but this jealousy tends to reduce after the baby is a year old. However, with more complicated family forms sibling rivalry can also exist between the children of parents who enter a new partnership. This can be especially the case where the mother has been a single parent, either through divorce or widowhood and starts a new relationship where there are existing children. The theory behind sibling rivalry is that children are competing for love and other resources – such as presents and treats – from their mother. Children can also feel that one parent has a favourite.

KEY TERM

Sibling – a sibling is your brother or sister and this may include stepbrothers and stepsisters.

Blended families

Family relationships can be quite complicated, especially when members have separated or made new relationships.

> **DISCUSSION**
>
> Children from a marriage may find it difficult to cope when their parents divorce and find new partners. Both men and women may find it difficult to get on with their partner's children from a previous relationship. The children of widowed parents are often very protective and can be suspicious of a new partner or step-parent.
>
> Step-families account for about 6% of all families with dependent children. Children usually stay with their mothers after a partnership breaks down.
>
> Relationships between parents, children and siblings can have positive effects, but they can also have negative effects.

> **KEY TERM**
>
> **Blended families** – the original adult partners have children and then separate or divorce and then form new partnerships, which may include children from earlier relationships.

> **ACTIVITY**
>
> Identify the negative and positive effects from the following examples of family life.
>
> 1. Surinder (age 8) lives with her parents and grandparents in West London in a small flat above the family business.
> 2. Merya (age 14) lives with her mother and older brother. Each weekend she goes to stay with her father and his new girlfriend.
> 3. James (age 6) is the youngest of four brothers who are aged 8, 10, and 12.
> 4. Susan (age 30) has just had her first baby. Her mother and mother-in-law are delighted at this event and cannot wait to give Sue the benefit of their advice.
> 5. Margaret is 75 years-of-age and lives on her own. Her son and daughter are married with their own families, but they live in the same area. They see their mother once a week and can help in emergencies. Margaret wishes she could see more of her grandchildren.

We can see from these examples that family relationships are formed:

- between parents
- between parents or step-parents and children
- between children
- between other relatives.

Friendships

Friendships are important social relationships that we choose to establish with other people because we share interests, or because we like each other. There is an emotional connection between friends, although it may not be as deep as in families. However, we all know the saying 'you can choose your friends but you cannot choose your family', and not everybody has a close relationship with their family. Friends can have close personal relationships, where they can talk about problems and receive emotional support, but we can also have more superficial relationships with people we would not identify as friends. Examples of this type of relationship could be neighbours, members of a church or social group, people

CASE STUDY 2 – Mary

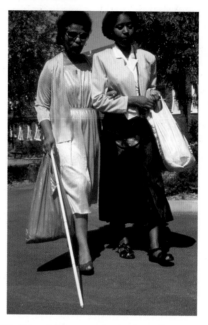

Figure 1.23 Friendships can last a long time

Mary (age 55) is blind. She was premature (born early) and as a result was blind. When she was 18-months-old she was sent to a residential home for blind children. When she was 11 Mary went to another residential Blind School. Mary says that her mother was very sad that her daughter had to live away from home and she only returned home for the holidays. Mary trained as a typist and she is now living in a flat on her own. She still keeps in touch with friends she made when she was at the Blind School. Mary has never married. She has friends who have married and have children. She says her friends are very important to her, as she has known them most of her life. Some of her friends are blind but others are sighted.

we see regularly and may chat to. In this type of relationship, you would not discuss personal matters.

As we have seen with Mary's story, close friendships can last a long time. Even if we change schools, move house, change jobs or get married, we will still keep some of our friends.

ACTIVITY

1. Make a list of your childhood friends (at primary school or in your local area). How many of these do you still see?
2. Which of your current friends do you think you will still be friendly with in 10 years time? Why do you think these friendships will last?

Intimate personal and sexual relationships

In early adulthood most people become interested in developing intimate relationships that may lead to stable partnerships and children. Many magazines, books and newspaper articles give advice on how to develop relationships. We have all seen letters in problem pages of magazines and television programmes on relationship difficulties. Close personal relationships can offer emotional support, as well as being a way of expressing our feelings sexually.

Working relationships

Work relationships are usually with people who are not members of our biological family and whose connection with us is more short-term. Work relationships are said to be secondary relationships for the following reasons:

- interaction between people is limited to work situations
- there are clear rules about how the relationship should be conducted
- there are clearly defined social roles (e.g. employer/worker, teacher/student).

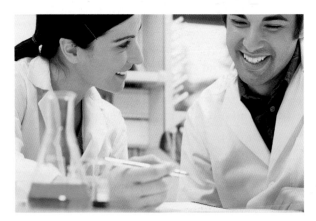

Figure 1.24 Work relationships can provide useful support

Relationships at work can be formal or informal. Formal relationships are those that are based on the work situation, and usually there is a power relationship (between the boss and employee, or the teacher and student). However, fellow workers may have informal relationships, which may be very important if the job is stressful or boring.

We can see in the example below that Louise has different relationships with colleagues, customers and her boss.

CASE STUDY 3 – Louise

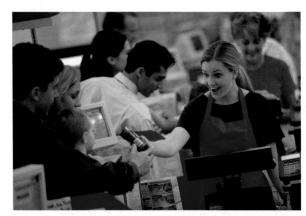

Figure 1.25 Louise at work

(continued)

> **CASE STUDY 3 – (continued)**
>
> Louise (age 16) is a student at a local college, but she works one evening and all day Saturday at a local supermarket on the till. Several other part-timer workers are also students, and they chat when they have their coffee break. At Christmas they went out for a meal at a local pub. Louise finds the work boring, but she needs the money. She says that the best thing about the job is the people that she works with. Her boss, Neil, told her off last week for being rude to a customer. Some customers are regulars who come to her till and have a chat. Louise enjoys this as it breaks the routine, but Neil told her she cannot do this too much if they are busy, as other customers start complaining.

Do you have a part-time job? What type of relationships do you have at work and do they affect how you feel about yourself? If we are being constantly put down by the boss or ignored by fellow workers, this can have a negative effect on how we feel about the job and also how we feel about ourselves. We all need to feel valued and appreciated, and it is important that employers show recognition of our efforts.

Most jobs have job descriptions that form the basis of the formal contract between the worker and employer. These state the duties of the job. However, jobs that are based on formal relationships alone would become very unfulfilling for the worker.

Members of professional groups, such as teachers and doctors, have clearly defined standards of behaviour towards their students or patients, and these are formal guidelines that need to be followed. If not, the professional may be disciplined and lose their job. Examples of this would be teachers who use their powerful position to have unlawful sexual relationships with their pupils, or doctors who have sexual relationships with their patients.

The importance of the effect of relationships on the six life stages

Erikson (1904–94) was a German psychologist who developed a theory about personal development throughout a person's lifetime. He felt that the relationships an individual has during childhood and later years affected their growth and development.

Table 1.14 outlines the key ideas. Erikson identified eight key life stages, but for this unit his eight-stage model has been adapted to fit the six stages discussed in this book. You can look for more about Erikson's model on the Internet.

Life stage	Crisis stage	Key relationships	Key activities	Positive outcome	Negative outcome
Infancy 0–2	Trust versus mistrust	Mother, family members	Feeding, being comforted, toilet training	Hope and drive	Withdrawal
Early childhood 3–8	Using initiative and becoming independent versus shame and doubt	Parents, teachers, friends,	Developing social skills, going to school/ nursery, making friends	Purpose and direction, confidence. Self-control 'fitting in'	Inhibition, difficulty making friends, lack of confidence

Table 1.14 The outcomes from relationships at six Key Stages in Life (adapted from Erikson)

Life stage	Crisis stage	Key relationships	Key activities	Positive outcome	Negative outcome
Adolescence 9–18	Identity versus role confusion	Peers, friends, social groups	Developing beliefs, interests and skills	Fidelity (loyalty) and devotion	Anti-social behaviour, criminal activities, fanatical views
Early adulthood 19–45	Intimacy versus isolation	Lovers, friends, work colleagues, intimate relationships, with partner and children	Commitment to others, a long-term relationship (marriage). Developing a career, becoming a parent	Feeling part of society and of a family in which the intimate relationship is mutually supportive	Isolation, social withdrawal, feeling excluded. Promiscuous behaviour. Poor self-esteem
Middle adulthood 46–65	Generative versus stagnant	Relationships with partners, children, the wider family circle, friends	Parenting teenagers, caring for older family members, coming to the end of a working life, doing voluntary work, 'giving back' to the community	Pride in life achievements and the achievements of family members, giving and caring, concern about global issues (such as global warming, or wars	Disinterested in life, 'stuck in a rut' miserable, depressed and isolated
Later adulthood 65+	Integrity versus despair	Family members, friends	Becoming a grandparent, leisure activities that stimulate, keeping up with friends	Feeling at peace with oneself and the world. Accepting one's death	Feeling that life has been unfair, wanting to turn the clock back, withdrawal from life, miserable and anti-social

Table 1.14 (continued)

DISCUSSION

Look at Table 1.14. You can see that this model seems to be based on people who have a partner and have children, but we know that not everyone falls into this category. You may know people who are in later adulthood and are single, have lots of friends and a good job. The other problem with this model is that it assumes that you move from one stage to the other at a certain age, but we all know that some people in their teens seem to behave in a very adult way, whereas some people in their twenties behave in a childish way. This model was developed in the 20th century and we know there have been great changes in that time. So what use is this model? It may be used to identify problems in clients we meet in health and social care. We can see that the early experiences of infancy and childhood can affect an individual for the rest of their life.

The effects of life events on personal development

We have already seen that life events impact on human growth and development. Life events can be expected or unexpected.

Relationship changes

Marriage

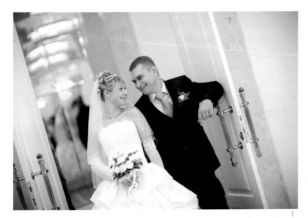

Figure 1.26 Marriage

Marriage is a life event that is celebrated by many people each year. Marriage involves a major change in personal development, especially a first marriage. The roles of the married couple change. Instead of being part of their birth families, they are now separate from their parents, and their main emotional and psychological commitment is to each other. As well as changing the relationship between the parents and the new couple, new relationships are also formed between the in-laws, who become part of the wider family network. In some cases, the married couple may have to move away from their parents because of work or housing, and this will make the couple very dependent on each other for support.

Living with a partner (cohabitation)

Many people are choosing to live with someone rather than get married. Some people live together before they get married, so we can see living together as a predictable event. Because there is usually no formal legal arrangement between couples who live together, this may cause stress on the couple, especially if they have children. Family members may disapprove of what they see as 'living in sin'. The couple themselves may see the arrangement as temporary, and this may lead to feelings of insecurity. Although many people live together very happily and see marriage as 'a piece of paper they don't need', other people may feel that if their partner is unwilling to make a commitment of marriage to them, they are not important to them, and this can lead to feelings of low self-esteem. Because they don't feel secure in the relationship, they can't relax and this affects their personal development.

Table 1.15 shows the numbers of people cohabiting by marital status in 2006.

Great Britain	Numbers in %			
	Single	**Widowed**	**Divorced**	**Separated**
Men				
Cohabiting[2]	22	2	34	23
Not cohabiting	78	98	66	77
All men	100	100	100	100
Women				
Cohabiting[2]	27	8	24	9
Not cohabiting	73	92	76	91
All women	100	100	100	100

1 Aged 16 to 59. See Appendix, Part 2: General Household Survey. Includes those who describe themselves as separated but were, in a legal sense, still married.
2 Includes a small number of same sex cohabiting.
Source: General Household Survey (Longitudinal), Office for National Statistics.
Table 1.15 People cohabiting: by marital status 2006[1]

ACTIVITY

1. Look at Table 1.15 and identify the main patterns you can see.

CASE STUDY 3 – Karl and Charlotte

Karl and Charlotte have been going out together for three years, since they met when they were in the Sixth Form. Both their families approve of the relationship, but Charlotte's mother keeps making remarks like, 'The neighbours are wondering when you are going to get married', and 'Your Gran thinks it's time Karl made an honest woman of you'. Unknown to their families, Karl and Charlotte have been looking at flats in their area, as they are thinking of renting a place together. Charlotte is nearing the end of her nursing training, and Karl has been offered promotion in the council, where he works in the housing department. They both feel they don't want to have children for a while – Charlotte is on the pill, and they are not sure about getting married, as they are still only 21-years-old. They want to live together and see how it works out, but they are dreading telling their parents.

Imagine you are a friend of theirs. How would you put forward arguments for and against them living together, rather than getting married?

Birth of children

Although the birth rate is falling in the UK, many people still expect to have children, whether they are married or not. Parenthood involves a major change in a person's life, with the additional pressures of responsibility and money worries. It is often said that once a couple become parents, they become adults. Although many people find having a child a wonderful experience, it can also be very demanding, especially for the woman. In spite of ideas about the 'new man', most women find they take on the main responsibility for child care.

Parents also need to decide on how to bring up the child; whether both parents can continue to work; how child care can be arranged. Other family members may also be involved, especially grandparents who may give conflicting advice, or criticise how child care is being managed.

Parenthood is often described as a '24-hour-a-day, 365-days-a-year job, with no time off, no pay and little recognition'. Mothers may find it difficult to make the change from going to work, going out socially and doing things on the spur of the moment, to looking after a demanding baby, a reduced social life and less money to spend. If the mother had a difficult pregnancy and birth, she may also feel that she has lost her figure; that no one, including her husband, will find her attractive any more, and that staying at home affects her self-confidence. Lack of sleep may affect her energy levels and she may be depressed.

Although having a baby can be a positive, enjoyable experience which can make a woman feel fulfilled, it can also feel rather a burden for both partners.

The father may feel that his partner's attention is focused on the baby and that he is ignored, so this can affect his self-image.

Death of partner

When a couple have been together for a long time and have children and grandchildren, it may be very difficult when one of them dies. Women are said to cope better with the death of their husband as they may have had to adapt to many changes in their lives – giving up work, raising children, going back to work and being at home. They also tend to have a wider group of friends who can support them at this difficult time. If you have been used to being a couple for many years it is hard to get used to being on your own, but for men it can be harder.

Death of a friend or relative

Although we know that we will all die, death can still have a great impact on our personal development. We expect older relatives to die before we do, and we know that we are likely to see the deaths of our parents and grandparents. In the UK, death is still seen as a subject many people prefer not to talk about, although death is marked by funeral services and rituals where the person's life is celebrated. Death of an older family member can be seen as a release, especially if they have been ill for a long time, but the death of this person can leave a gap in the lives of the people who are left. It is natural to feel sad and to miss the person.

Research has shown that if there was a good relationship between the person who died and the bereaved person, then sadness will gradually be replaced with acceptance, and the good memories of the past. If there was a difficult relationship, the person left may feel guilty and find it difficult to get over the death. In this case, professional help may be needed. When our older family members die, we then take on the roles of leading the family.

Divorce

When a couple meet, fall in love and get married, they decide they are going to stay together for the rest of their lives and make vows to that effect. They do not intend to get divorced. The breakdown of the marriage and the process of divorce have an emotional impact on the couple. When the couple have children, these problems are increased, as decisions will have to be made about who will have care of the children. Separate accommodation and income arrangements will have to be made. Dealing with solicitors and courts can also be stressful. The grandparents will also be affected. If the couple finds new partners, this will bring in other relationships. Both men and women can feel guilty and have a sense of failure over the ending of the marriage. The woman may have to make major adjustments to her life, if she has to work full-time to support the family, taking responsibility for money and running a household that she had previously left to her husband, or shared in the past. Divorce can be seen as a challenge, and some women find it a positive challenge and develop their confidence and ability to hold down a job. Others may feel rejected by their husbands. They feel they will never find another partner and feel lonely and depressed. Research has shown that divorced men are more likely to remarry, but that second marriages are more likely to fail. Divorced men are more likely to become ill, and turn to alcohol and other forms of addiction. Figure 1.27 shows the divorce and remarriage rates. Identify the main patterns you see.

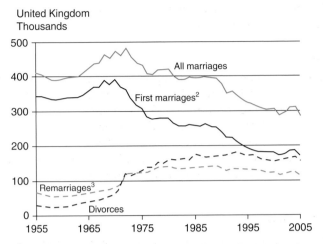

United Kingdom
Thousands

[1] Divorce data from 1955 to 1970 are for Great Britain only. Divorce becam legal in Northern Ireland from 1969. Includes annulments.
[2] For both partners.
[3] For one or both partners.

Figure 1.27 Divorce and remarriage rates

Physical changes that affect our personal development

Puberty

Adolescence and puberty can be disturbing times. Girls and boys can develop secondary sexual characteristics at different times. It can be difficult for a 15-year-old boy who is shorter than the rest of his classmates, or for a girl who started her periods in junior school and found there were no facilities for the disposal of sanitary protection. The development of breasts, or the lack of them, can cause feelings of inadequacy and lack of self-confidence. Spots, braces on the teeth, and sudden growth spurts can all be disturbing and confusing. It is important that the young person is given positive support and reassurance during this time. Adolescence is a difficult stage between childhood and adulthood. It is important that young people feel valued and respected so that they have a positive self-concept. This provides a firm basis for adjustment to adult life.

The menopause

Just as puberty is an expected change, so is the menopause. This marks the end of a woman's reproductive life phase, and can be seen as a positive change, as it means that anxiety about unwanted pregnancy is removed. It can also be seen as a negative time, when a woman may feel physically unattractive as her hormones change, and some of the physical symptoms can be unpleasant – night sweats, increased anxiety, dry skin and headaches. Although the GP can prescribe effective medication to assist the physical changes, it is important that the woman maintains a positive self-image. Her children may be older and she may have more time for herself and her husband. She may be able to take up interests she never had time to do before.

Accident or illness leading to disability

Some people are born with or inherit physical or learning disabilities. Others acquire a disability as a result of accident or illness, for example being involved in a car accident.

CASE STUDY 4 – Mark

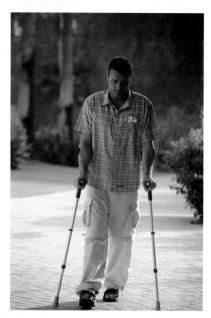

Figure 1.28 Mark

Mark's story.

Mark is now 35 years old.

'I was 28 and I had just got married. I used to play rugby on Saturdays. Some days I noticed I was seeing double, but I put it down to overdoing things and getting tired. I then started getting pins and needles in my arm and leg on the left side. One day I got out of bed and nearly fell over; my balance seemed to go. I went to see the GP. He referred me to the specialist. After a lot of tests I was told I had multiple sclerosis (MS). I was absolutely gutted. I had just got a new job teaching in a school in the West Country, and we had been thinking about starting a family. The head teacher was really helpful, but my wife found it all too much and we split up soon after I was diagnosed – probably my fault, as I became very sorry for myself and difficult to live with.

Since I was diagnosed I have had some flare ups when I can hardly move and I have spent time in hospital for assessment. My car has been adapted so I don't need to use the foot pedals. I have moved into a ground-floor flat. I am still working full time at the moment. I can get about the school using a stick, but I might need to use a wheelchair at some point.

The worst thing about the disease is that you don't know how fast it will progress. I might be like I am at the moment for a while. I look at rugby on the television and I really miss playing. I have found the adjustment has been really difficult, as I was so fit and independent. I have a new girl friend now, and that has made a tremendous difference. If anything, I feel the experience of MS has made me more aware of the importance of enjoying life while I can and making the most of every day. I couldn't have coped without my friends.'

People who become disabled have to adapt their lifestyle to cope with the disability. We can see from Mark's story that even very negative events can be a means to achieve personal development. Not everyone may have Mark's resilience, and adapting to serious illness and disability can be a challenge.

Changes in life circumstances are other events that can affect our personal development

Starting school

This is one of the first predictable life events for all children. Beginning primary school is a turning point in children's lives. It means that the child is going to leave the support of parents and the home setting, and move into the wider social setting of school, where new patterns of behaviour will occur. Many children (and their parents) find the first day of school very frightening. Many schools recognise this and have a system where children start off with a half day and then move to a full day at school. With more nursery classes attached to primary schools, children become used to the school. The move to secondary school can be more difficult, especially if the child has not managed to get into the school preferred by their parents. Children need the support of parents, brothers and sisters, and teachers to cope successfully with this life change.

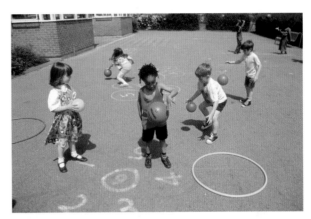
Figure 1.29 Young children in a primary school

Starting further education

Many teenagers find that they don't want to stay on in the Sixth Form or perhaps the school does not offer the courses they want to do.

CASE STUDY 5 – Ella

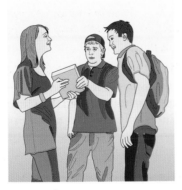
Figure 1.30 Ella at college

I was at an all girls' school and I found that it was a very academic school and unless you wanted to be a doctor or a lawyer after university the teachers weren't really interested in you. I wasn't sure what I wanted to do either, but I knew I wanted to leave at 16. I went to an open evening at

(continued)

CASE STUDY 5 – (continued)

the local college. It seemed huge but the teachers were friendly. I knew someone who had been there and had done the health and social care course and she really enjoyed it, especially the work experience. She is at a university doing a degree in nursing now. I found the first term was quite hard – you were treated like an adult and expected to get on with your work. It took me a while to make friends, but now I am really pleased that I made the change. I feel I have grown up a lot since I came here.

Relocation

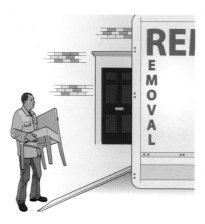

Figure 1.31 Moving house

Relocation means moving from one area to another. It could be moving from one county in England to another, or it could be moving abroad.

Moving house has been seen as one of the most stressful events in one's life and moving usually is as a result of a change in circumstances such as:

- getting married
- getting divorced
- having children
- taking a new job in another part of the country (or abroad)
- being unable to cope with a large house.

Moving house can involve making a decision about where to live, the finances that are available and signing up to a mortgage. Moving house can also involve moving from close friends and family; in older children it may involve changing schools and leaving their friends. If the move is to another country there could be language or cultural differences that the family or person will have to adapt to.

Entering the employment market

Starting work represents the transition to adulthood; it means that we have to be responsible, and behave as independent adults. However, although work can be exciting and stimulating, it can also be boring. All jobs can be repetitive. As part of our personal development we need to be able to adapt to the demands made on us by work. We develop skills, such as time management and attention to detail, which may be very important. We also need to develop social skills, as in most jobs we will be working with people as colleagues or as clients.

The development of these interpersonal skills is all part of our personal development.

Promotion

In many work situations there are opportunities to get promoted to more senior jobs with more responsibilities. These jobs often mean you have to have more training to get more qualifications. You may work longer hours. Perhaps you were a member of a team, but in your new role you may have to be their boss. If several people applied from the department for the job, they may resent you for being successful. Some people decide they do not want promotion because they don't have the confidence to go for it and they are happy keeping to the job they know well. Whether you are seen as a 'go-getter' or someone who likes the' easy option', can affect your self-concept, as we have already seen that the way people react to us can have an important effect on our self-esteem.

Retirement

Although we may spend much of our life in work, the time spent in retirement is increasing as we live longer. Some people see retirement as a release from the daily grind and routine of work, but some people see retirement as a time of anxiety. They feel they have lost their identity, especially if their job was very important to them and had high status. Women who have spent time bringing up a family may worry that they will not have enough money to manage, as they may not have much in the way of a pension. We still have to eat, maintain a house or flat, keep warm and pay the bills when we retire, even though we are not working. Many retired people miss the social contact that they had at work. If retirement can be a time to do those things that were not possible when we were working, then this helps personal development, but if people experience poverty and loneliness, this has a very negative effect on a person's self-image.

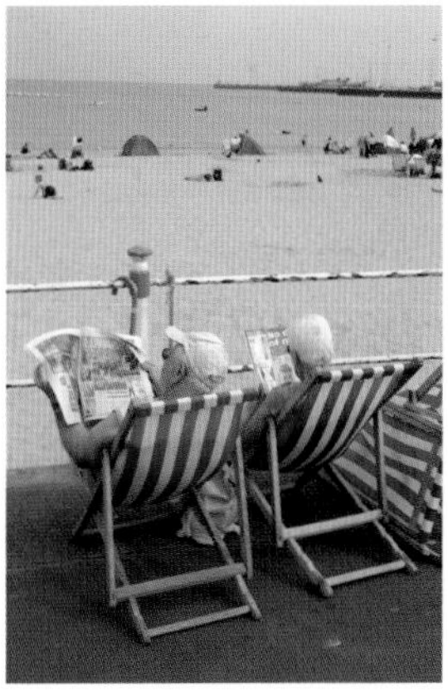

Figure 1.32

Redundancy

Redundancy happens when an employer decides that a job no longer exists and the worker is given notice of redundancy, losing their job through no fault of their own. This can happen when two firms merge, or there is an economic recession. Redundancy can have a great effect on an individual's self-esteem, as well as affecting their income. People who have been made redundant can feel worthless, especially if they have been in the company for many years and

---

CASE STUDY 6 – Peter

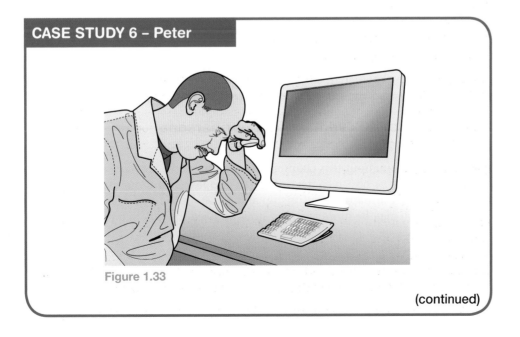

Figure 1.33

(continued)

CASE STUDY 6 – (continued)

'I had worked for the company for 17 years in their office in the City. There had been a lot of changes when we were taken over by another firm, but redundancy had never been mentioned.

I went into the office as usual on the Monday and was called into the manager's office. I was told that changes were being made and that new I.T. systems were being introduced. They felt that as I was 50 I would find it difficult to cope with the changes and my old job would not exist any more.

I was asked to clear my desk and be out of the office by lunchtime. I felt really ill. I couldn't believe what was happening. I had worked really hard for the firm for all those years. I was worried about the family – we had four children, and three were still at school. My wife worked part-time. I went home and went to bed because I felt so awful. I had to tell my wife when she got in from work. I had made a lot of friends in the firm and in the City, but when I rang them they didn't want to talk to me. They said they would look out for a job for me, but they never rang me back. I wrote 60 letters to people I knew asking for a job, but I wasn't successful. In the end, I found another job at a smaller company on lower pay, but I shall never feel secure again. You never know – it might happen again.'

worked hard. They can wonder what the point was of all the years they spent working, if they are then told they have to leave. In some cases, the decision to make workers redundant can happen overnight.

We can see from Peter's story that redundancy can have a severe and lasting effect on someone's self-image. However, some people have used redundancy as an opportunity to have a fresh start, returning to study or training for a new career.

Unemployment

Unemployment can happen at any time. At the moment, many young people leave school and cannot find work; this could be because they live in an area where the factories and other places of employment have closed, or it could be because they do not have the skills and qualifications needed.

How do these life events affect our personal development?

We have seen throughout this chapter that the life events we have discussed can have negative or positive effects. We can also learn from our experiences. If we have had an unhappy relationship and move on to form a new relationship, we may be more aware of how we need to work at a relationship and how we may be successful in the future. If we are in a job we find boring, we may fulfil ourselves in a voluntary group that give us satisfaction – using skills we don't use at work. If you have had a difficult teenage experience yourself, you may be able to relate more easily to young people who are having a hard time, and offer them support. All the life events we experience can be used in a positive way.

CASE STUDY 7 – Helen

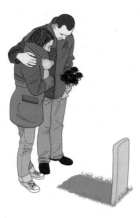

Figure 1.34

Helen had been married for three years when she had her first baby – Teresa. Helen found it difficult to cope with the new baby and things became even worse when the baby died unexpectedly when she was 3-weeks-old. The police had to investigate her death, and Helen and Mike (her husband) felt very guilty and upset and they had no one to talk to. Teresa had died from natural causes – cot death. The years went by and Helen and Mike had four more children, but they never forgot Teresa. Helen found out there is now an organisation – the Foundation for Sudden Infant Death (FSID) – that supports families who have experienced a cot death and Helen trained to be a befriender. She has befriended many parents who have had a cot death and they all say to her how helpful it is to talk to someone who has had the same experience. Sometimes Helen can feel sad when the parents ask her about Teresa, but usually she feels she has been able to help people just by listening to their story.

We can see from Teresa's story that our experiences may be used in a positive way. Many health and social care workers have had the experience of being in care themselves, and this can help them understand their clients' problems

How can we manage change in our lives?

We all have to manage change in our lives from the point at which we first leave our mothers to go to play group to when we retire from an active life. With every stage in our lives we may feel regret at leaving behind certain experiences and people, but we need to move forward with confidence and hope to the next stage in our lives. This is where the Erikson model is useful, as we can see that each stage has its own problems, but we can make a difference to the outcome if we experience life in a positive way.

Support from partners, family and friends

Sometimes we may feel unable to cope with significant changes in our lives, such as bereavement, illness, disability or the breakdown of a relationship. As part of a close relationship with a partner – perhaps in marriage – we would expect to have mutual emotional support. Family members can also provide support, but again, relationships in some families can be difficult and it may be easier to discuss personal problems with a close friend. As we have already found on page 20, research shows that those people who have 10 friends are more likely to be happier than those with few friends. However, there can be problems in discussing difficulties with close family or friends. They tend to see us in a good light and may say what they think we want to hear. For example, if a girl says to her friend, 'Does my bum look big in this?' the friend is more likely to say she looks fine because she knows if she is honest they may not continue to be friends! For this reason, it may be more useful to discuss problems with professionals who see you in a less emotional way.

Professional support

GPs are reporting an increase in advising patients who have social problems rather than medical problems. A patient may see the GP because they are not sleeping, but by talking to the patient the GP realises that the problem is about work, family situations or other difficulties. Most surgeries can now refer patients to a counsellor who will see the patient for about six sessions. On the NHS, this service is free, but patients can also refer themselves to private counsellors, although they would have to pay.

CASE STUDY 8 – Diane

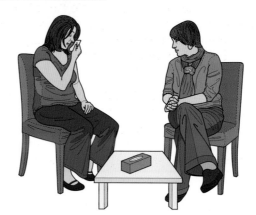

Figure 1.35 Diane

Diane works as a counsellor in a private practice. Her clients are referred to her by local doctors and other health professionals, but she is also recommended by clients she has helped. Diane sees a wide range of people who have experienced difficulties in their lives. She says that she sees her role as helping people to look at the situation that is upsetting them so that they can move on with their lives.

Diane is a psycho-dynamic counsellor. She knows she cannot change the things that have happened to people, but she can help them look at the problem in a different way. She finds many of the problems people have in coping with life, relate to experiences they had in childhood that have left them feeling unhappy and unloved.

We can see from Diane's work that Eriksson's theories can still be applied to supporting people nowadays.

There are many professionals who can help with family problems related to child care. The health visitor can offer advice and support. Social workers can also offer support in a range of problems, especially related to illness, disability, poverty and unemployment. Support can also be offered by psychologists, who offer a range of services such as one-to-one therapy or group therapy to people who may have difficulties coping with issues in their lives. Other specialists can include physiotherapists and occupational therapists, for example.

Community, voluntary and faith based services

There are many charities and organisations that offer support. We have already discussed the support given by FSID to bereaved parents. The charity Cruse can offer support to bereaved people; the Citizens Advice Bureau can give advice on people's rights and benefits; Age Concern can offer support to older people; Relate offers support for people who are having problems with their marriage or partnerships. Local churches and religious groups can also offer support and guidance.

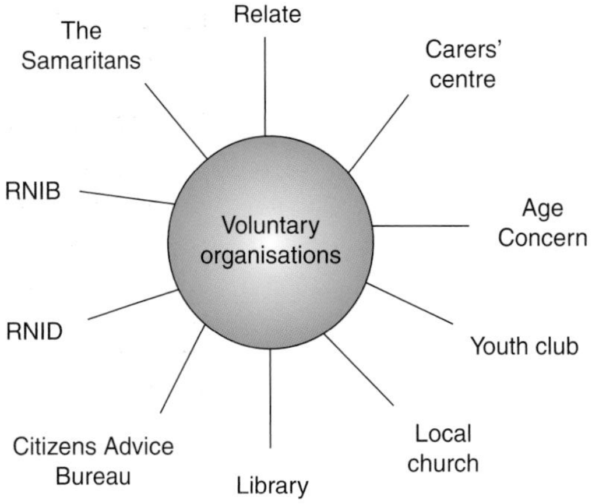

Many of the professional and voluntary groups that offer support will be listed in local directories or in the library. The internet gives details of organisations that give support to particular groups. Organisations such as the Royal Institute for the Deaf (RNID) and the Royal Institute for the Blind (RNIB) offer support to disabled people and have a website.

Figure 1.36 Diagram of organisations that offer support

Self-help groups are a further source of support. No Panic is a self-help group that was set up to support people who experience panic attacks. Panic attacks can occur following life changes, and finding support from a local group can be very helpful. You can find a full list of self-help groups on the following web site: www.self-help.org.uk

As we can see, we may all experience difficulties during our lives. Expected and unexpected events may force us to cope with change. Our reactions to these events can affect our health and well-being, so it is important that we find ways to cope. If we are unable to adjust to changes, this may result in serious physical, psychological and social problems which will affect our personal development and well-being.

GLOSSARY

Absolute poverty – a lack of resources sufficient to maintain a healthy existence

Abuse – treating people badly, either physically or emotionally

Chronic condition – a disease of long duration involving very slow changes. It often starts very gradually

Cohabitation – a couple living together who are not married or in a civil partnership

Culture – shared values based on beliefs, practice, dress, language, diet and religion

Discrimination – the unfair treatment of a person, or group, because of a negative view of some, or all, of their characteristics (could be based on ethnicity, gender or age)

Disease – a specific condition of ill health, identified as an actual change on the surface or inside some part of the body

GLOSSARY – (continued)

Emotional health – concerned with being able to express feelings such as fear, joy, grief, frustration and anger. It also includes the ability to cope with anxiety, stress, and depression

Ethnicity – a shared identity which comes from a common culture, religion or tradition

Gender – the psychological and social development of male and female roles in a society

Homophobia – fear and hatred of homosexuals

Ideal self – the type of person you would most like to be

Identity – self image; how you see yourself and what you know about yourself

Illness – the subjective state of feeling unwell (i.e. how people feel) (Compare with Disease and Sickness)

Income – the sum of all earnings of a household or individual in a given period of time

Intellectual health – this is concerned with the ability to think clearly and rationally. It is closely linked to emotional and social health.

Material possessions – the things a person owns

Menopause – when women stop menstruating

Nuclear family – family consisting of one woman and one man with dependent children

Physical health – concerned with the physical functioning of the body. It is the easiest aspect of health to measure.

Poverty – lack of resources helping you to be healthy

Primary relationship – close relationship based on kinship, marriage, adoption, friendship or blood ties

Redundancy – when work or a job no longer exists for the worker who is then made unemployed

Relative poverty – a lack of resources (income) sufficient to achieve a standard of living considered acceptable in a society

Role model – an example of behaviour or achieved status in society that is seen as good

Secondary relationship – more distant or formal relationship that may be short term

Self-concept – how you see yourself as a separate individual

Self-image (identity) – how you see yourself and what you know about yourself

Self-esteem – the value you place on yourself

Self-fulfilling prophecy – a belief that things turn out as you predict because people behave in such a way as to bring about the prediction- usually to do with behaviour

Sibling – brother or sister

Sickness – reported illness; involves being treated by a professional and becoming a medical statistic

Social health – this is concerned with the ability to relate to others and to form relationships

Social role – the way you behave in certain situations, such as a student, nurse, etc

GLOSSARY – (continued)

Socialisation – the way you learn as a child how to fit into society using the social skills and values of that society

Status – your social position related to others so may be high or low; linked to factors such as wealth, income, social class, job, age and appearance

Stereotype – a simplified general image about a particular group of people, e.g. 'they all do that'

Wealth – the extent of an individual's or household's possessions and resources

Working relationship – relationship based in working environment that is more distant or formal

CHAPTER 2

Exploring Health, Social Care and Early Years Provision

CHAPTER CONTENT

This chapter will help you learn about:
- the range of care needs of the major client groups in health, social care and early years
- how health care, social care and early years services are accessed
- the barriers that can exist for access to services
- how health, social care and early years services are provided
- the workers in health, social care and early years services
- the care values that underpin service provider interaction

This unit is assessed under controlled conditions. You will need to provide one report, which will be based on an investigation of the needs of one service user and how these needs are met by service providers and care practitioners.

In this book you will find many words are used that you may not have seen before. Throughout the chapter you will find that important words are defined. They will also be included in the glossary at the end of the book.

In order to help you with the assessment, it may be helpful if you collect newspaper articles, leaflets and other materials related to health, social care and early years services in a folder that you could use in discussions with your groups, or in the assessment.

Throughout the book there will be exercises and activities to help you work through the material.

The range of care needs of major client groups

KEY TERM

Service user – anyone who uses health and social care services.

The groups who may use health, social care and early years services

The groups who may use health, social care and early years services could be divided into the following groups.

Infants (0–2 years)

A baby is defined as being aged under 1-year-old. In the first year of life a baby is very dependent on adults, usually parents, to provide their needs. During this first year, a baby develops from being totally dependent to becoming mobile and developing the ability to interact with others and to play.

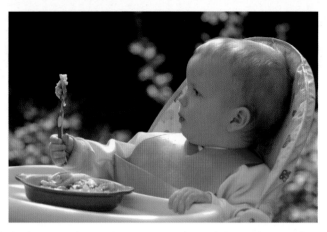

Figure 2.1 A baby has certain needs

Children (3–8 years)

As young children grow older they are able to do more for themselves, but they are still dependent on other people to look after them. Children experience many changes as they grow – going to playgroups, nursery and infants school. They may have a new brother or sister. They will make friends outside the family and develop new skills, such as leaning to ride a tricycle and to read.

Adolescents (9–18 years)

Adolescence and the teenage years are seen as a period of rapid growth and development and emotional change.

ACTIVITY

Perhaps you are a teenager yourself. If not, imagine being a 14-year-old today. Make a list of all the good things about being 14. Then make a list of all the bad things about being 14. You could compare your list with other people in your class. How are they similar and how are they different? Are there differences depending on whether you are a girl or a boy? Some people find that parents are stricter with their daughters than with their sons.

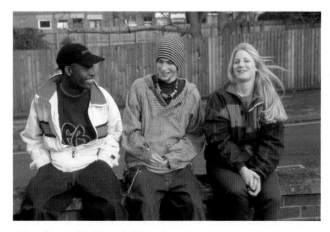

Figure 2.2 The transition from child to adulthood

Table 2.1 shows the answers given by youth workers who were given this exercise.

Positive	Negative

Meeting new people
Trying out new experiences:
  – drinking alcohol
  – smoking
  – going out with friends
  – belonging to a group
More personal freedom
Having first girlfriend/boyfriend
Trying out new clothes, hairstyles, make-up
Having first job – earning money
Feeling grown up
Feeling independent
Deciding what to do in free time
Close friendships
Excited about the future
Sense of personal identity
	Feeling shy and awkward, meeting new people
	Having spots/weight problems
	Starting periods/voice breaking
	Physical changes: breasts, body hair
	Feeling lonely, isolated
	Parents don't understand you
	Not belonging to a group
	Worried about school work, bullying
	Not having a girlfriend/boyfiend
	Anxiety about sexuality
	Being treated like a child
	Too young to do some things, too old to do others
	Trouble with police, teachers
	Anxiety about the opposite sex
	Dislike of own appearance
	Using drugs, sniffing glue, getting drunk as a way of coping
	Depressed and anxious about the future
	Not sure of own identity

Table 2.1 Experience of being 14-years-old

Look at Table 2.1 and think about the needs that young people may have as a result of their experience of being 14. Although this can be an exciting time, young people can also experience confusion, sadness and anxiety.

The family may not be able to meet all the needs of this age group. Other health and care workers may need to be involved in supporting them. These could include school nurses, specialist workers dealing with drugs, sexual health and mental health problems.

Connexions is a government programme, aimed at meeting the needs of young people between the age of 13 and 19 as they approach adulthood.

ACTIVITY

Go to the Connexions website: www.connexions.gov.uk and look at the services provided. There will be a local service in your area. You should be able to find details about it in your school, youth club or library.

Adults

Adulthood can be divided into 3 groups: early, middle and later.

Early adulthood (normally seen as people aged between 19 and 45)

In this period there is quite a variety of activities that people undertake. Some people in this group may be at university or college; others may be developing a career; others may be married and having a family; some women may be single parents. Because of the diversity of the population in the UK nowadays, the experience of young people in this age group is very varied

Middle adulthood (could include people between the ages of 46 and 65)

In this period most people are establishing themselves and their families in both their personal lives and in their work situation. In a family with two parents and teenage children, both parents may work, but the parents can also be seen as an 'in-between group' who care for their older parents as well as caring for grandchildren.

Later adulthood (people over the age of 65)

In the UK nowadays the numbers of people over 65 are increasing. More people are celebrating their 100th birthday than ever before. This means that some social care professionals talk about the 'young old', as well as the older groups. Most people between the ages of 65 and 75 can still enjoy life, although they may be more likely to have chronic illnesses like asthma, arthritis or diabetes.

Because people are living longer in the UK and are in better health than in previous generations, it is difficult to give exact boundaries between these groups. You may have heard people say 'that 60 is the new 40'. If you look at old family photographs, you may notice that people seem to look quite old when they were in their 20s.

Becoming adult does not mean that we no longer have needs. Adults may have greater pressures put on them through work and family responsibilities, including the care of young and older family members. There can be additional pressures because of gender stereotyping, with women being seen as the natural carers in the family, although they may also be working, and men still being seen as the main breadwinner of the family, in spite of rising unemployment in traditional male jobs.

> **KEY TERM**
>
> Stereotype – a simplified general image about a particular group of people – they all do –, they all are –.

Individuals with specific needs

Many people have specific needs. According to the 2001 census about 20% of the UK adult population are disabled. That is about 11 million people. Disabilities can include:

- sensory disabilities – hearing, vision
- physical disabilities, which may affect mobility and could include cerebral palsy
- mental health problems, such as schizophrenia or depression
- learning disabilities, such as Downs Syndrome.

Some disabilities are inherited conditions such as Huntington's Chorea, where a faulty gene leads to the disabling condition.

Some disabilities are developmental conditions, where the foetus is affected in the womb in some way, such as if the mother contracts Rubella (German measles) and this can cause deafness and blindness.

Illness and accident are the main causes of disability occurring in those born without a disability. Road traffic accidents are the most common cause of accidents causing disability.

Physical, intellectual, emotional and social needs

In this section we will look at the differing Physical, Intellectual, Emotional and Social needs across the different needs of major client groups:

- Physical
- Intellectual
- Emotional
- Social

One way of remembering this is to use the word 'PIES' (see Chapter 1, pages 1–2).

Table 2.2 shows examples of how these needs could be grouped under these different categories.

Physical needs	Intellectual needs	Emotional needs	Social needs
Keeping warm, having a good diet, and taking exercise	Making use of your abilities	Being able to express feelings, joy, sadness	Developing relationships with others
Being safe	Using and developing language skills	Being able to cope with anxiety, depression and stress	Feeling part of a family/community
Being free from disease, illness and infection	Learning new skills	Feeling supported emotionally	Having friends
Keeping healthy	Doing stimulating work	Being respected as a person	Social interaction
Preventing ill-health, e.g by having immunisations	Developing written skills		Becoming independent
Maintaining personal hygiene	Developing IT skills		Developing effective communication
Using medication to keep healthy	Using leisure activities to develop skills		

Table 2.2 Examples of physical, intellectual, emotional and social needs grouped under different categories

Problems with grouping

You must remember that these different aspects of a person's needs are not separate but overlap and influence one another.

For example, if our social needs are met because of our contacts with friends and family, this can have a positive impact on our emotional well-being.

Another way of looking at our needs is to use Maslow's Hierarchy of Needs.

Abraham Maslow (1908–1970) was a psychologist. He believed that the purpose of life was personal growth. In his model you can see that there are different levels on the pyramid. Maslow believed that the basic needs of hunger, thirst, and warmth must be met before the higher needs can be achieved. However, the model has been criticised, as at different times of our lives certain needs may be more important. We have all read about a composer or writer, who spent all their time developing their skills but often did not eat enough or look after themselves physically, as they were so absorbed in their work and fulfilling their full potential.

At different stages of our lives our needs may change, and the type of support we need may also alter.

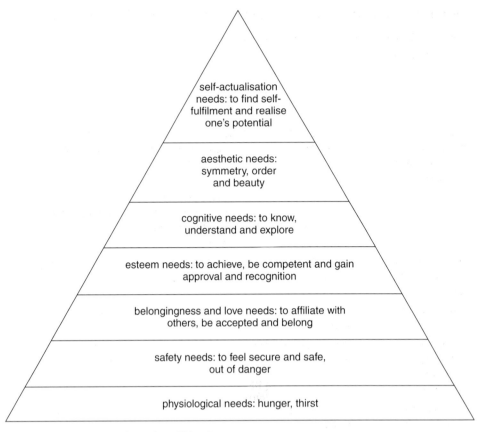

Figure 2.3 Maslow's Hierarchy of Needs

In this section we will look in more detail at the physical, intellectual, emotional and social needs of the following client groups:

- infants (0–2 years)
- early childhood (3–8 years)
- adolescents (9–18)
- young adults (19–45)
- middle aged adults (46–65)
- older people 66 years+
- people with specific needs.

Infants

An infant is defined as aged under 2-years-old. In the first year of life, a baby is very dependent on adults, usually parents, to provide their health, developmental and social care needs. During this first year, a baby develops from being totally dependent to becoming mobile, and developing the ability to interact with others and to play.

ACTIVITY

Look at Table 2.2 and identify the key needs that are relevant in the first year of life.

How would you make sure that these needs are met?

Physical needs

You may have included the following in your list:

- making sure the baby has the recommended immunisations
- keeping the baby away from sources of infection
- making sure that feeds and equipment used by the baby are clean
- keeping the baby warm
- dressing the baby in adequate clothing.

Intellectual needs

- using toys and interaction with the baby to develop their communications skills
- developing the baby's ability to play.

Emotional needs

Supporting and encouraging the child to try new experiences and reassuring them when they are anxious.

Social needs

Encouraging the baby to develop relationships with the wider family members and family friends.

Young children

As children grow older they are able to do more for themselves, but they are still dependent on other people to look after them. Children experience many changes as they grow, going to playgroups, nursery, and infants school. They may have a new brother or sister. They will make friends outside the family and develop new interests and new skills, such as learning to ride a tricycle.

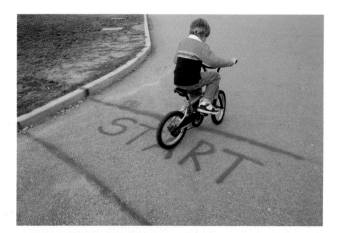

Figure 2.4 Thomas on his bike

CASE STUDY 1

Thomas, who is 7-years-old, attends the local primary school. He takes a packed lunch to school. Sometimes he goes to tea with a friend after school. At the weekends he plays football in a local group, and he likes to go swimming.

ACTIVITY

By the age of 7 most children have developed a range of skills, including reading and writing, and their language is well-established so they are able to communicate their feelings.

Look at Table 2.2 and decide which needs are most relevant to Thomas.

DISCUSSION

One of the key difficulties facing parents of young children is balancing the need to encourage independence and self-confidence, while making sure that risks to the child are reduced. Living with risk is part of life, and if we try to reduce all risk we can affect the positive development of a young child.

Physical needs

You may have included in your list immunisations, maintaining a healthy diet and lifestyle, and personal hygiene, such as encouraging children to wash their hands after using the toilet and before eating meals.

Intellectual needs

Thomas is developing intellectual skills at school by learning to read and write and use the computer. At home he may be read books, play board games and take part in other activities that meet his intellectual needs.

Emotional needs

Thomas is still very dependent on his family to support him emotionally, especially if he has a difficult day at school.

Social needs

The development of independence and social relationships is a very important part of growing up.

ACTIVITY

Look at the following examples of people of different ages. Identify the physical, intellectual, emotional and social needs they have. In your groups decide what they could do, or health and social care workers could do, to meet their needs

1. Shaziya is a 16-year-old student, working for her GCSEs. She feels very stressed and anxious all the time. Her best friend recently left the school and she feels no one really cares about her. Her mother is busy in her work. Shaziya has developed bad headaches.
2. Karl (17) has been in a relationship with Lindsay for a year now. They have decided to find out about contraception.
3. Helena (20) is a single parent. Her daughter (Sky) is 2-years-old. Helena is exhausted all the time as Sky never sleeps at night. Helena would like to go out with her friends and her neighbour has offered to babysit. Helena sometimes thinks she should never have had the baby; she never realized how difficult it would be and she feels very isolated.

(continued)

ACTIVITY – (continued)

4. Henry (55) had a bad pain in his chest. The hospital said he had suffered a heart attack. Henry has always been fit and active and he feels very depressed. He will have to take pills every day. He feels like an old man sitting in the house all day looking at TV, but he is nervous of doing anything in case he has another attack.
5. Mary (62) was a carer for her husband Frank for four years. He finally died of cancer recently. Mary feels very tired. Because Frank could not be left very often, she lost touch with most of her friends. She has two grown-up children and two grandchildren, but she feels 'they have their own lives now and they live far away'.

It is important that people's needs are met. What may happen to these people if their needs are not met?

DISCUSSION

1. Shaziya could start taking painkillers for her headaches; this could be dangerous. She may feel that no one is interested in her and this will affect her intellectual and emotional development; she may drop out of education. Shaziya could become increasingly isolated and could end up with depression.
2. Karl needs to decide with Lindsay what they should do. Perhaps they could go to a young people's clinic that will offer advice and contraception. Karl and Lindsay need to be made aware of sexually transmitted infections. If Lindsay became pregnant because they had not received advice, this could have an impact on both of them and could affect their physical, intellectual (if they have to drop their studies) emotional and social development.
3. Helena needs to be supported and helped – perhaps by a voluntary organization such as Homestart – to learn about child care and find out about child minding opportunities, in case she decides she wants to go back to work. If her needs were not met, this would have an impact on her relationship with her daughter; she may leave her daughter alone while she is out with her friends or she may physically harm her daughter. Helena's development will be affected physically, through lack of sleep; intellectually, if she feels unable to leave Sky and follow her own interests and develop new skills; emotionally, if she is having difficulty adapting to being a parent; and socially, as she is very isolated.
4. Henry may become isolated. He may take too much or too little medication. His health will suffer if he does no exercise so his health may get worse. Henry's development will be adversely affected in the following ways. Physically, if he takes no exercise; intellectually, if he has no interests or hobbies; emotionally, if he becomes isolated; and socially, if he withdraws from society.
5. Mary may become very depressed. It is very difficult for a carer to adjust to life without the person they cared for. Depression can cause a range of physical problems like headaches, feelings of panic, using

(continued)

DISCUSSION – (continued)

alcohol or smoking to relieve the misery. Mary's development will be affected: physically, if she does not rest and take care of her own health; intellectually, if she has no stimulating interests; emotionally, if she remains isolated; and socially, if she does not make an effort to make new friends or to get in touch with the friends she has.

We can see from these examples that it is very important that people's needs are met, otherwise worse problems can occur and their personal development is adversely affected.

Statistics show that more people are living into their eighties and nineties, and this client group may have particular needs. Physical ageing is a natural process and can result in declining physical ability, including loss of vision, and hearing and mobility problems.

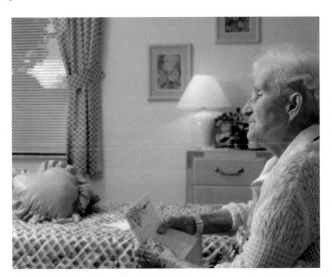

Figure 2.5 Older people have a range of needs

CASE STUDY 2 – Beatrice

Beatrice is a 90-year-old widow, who lives on her own in a three-bedroomed house. Her married daughter sees her every week. Beatrice has diabetes, and this has caused problems with her sight and also with ulcers on her leg. The local social services have organised a home help who comes weekly to clean the house; a shopper comes every fortnight to do her shopping. Beatrice is very independent and, although she has problems walking because of arthritis, she gets the local minibus service to the town once a week to collect her pension. Beatrice enjoys reading, but listening to the radio and watching television are becoming more difficult, as she is quite deaf. Many of her friends have died, and she has no contact with her neighbours.

What are Beatrice's needs? Can you group them under the headings used in Table 2.2?

Who can support Beatrice so that she can fulfil these needs?

What may happen to Beatrice if her needs are not met?

Although Beatrice has some clearly identified physical needs, such as the need to monitor her diabetes, we can see that her physical needs have an impact on all aspects of her life. If Beatrice cannot communicate easily because of her hearing problem, and cannot get out and about because of the arthritis, this affects her emotionally and socially. Many older people are not aware of financial benefits they are entitled to, and this can affect their physical, intellectual, emotional and social well-being. They worry about not being able to pay for heating and other bills so they do not eat properly or keep warm. They can become isolated with little social interaction. They lose interest in activities such as reading or doing puzzles.

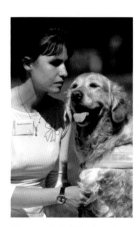

Figure 2.6 Disabled people have a range of needs

People with specific needs

People with disabilities make up about 20% of the population aged 16+, according to the 2001 census figures. As we have seen on page 65 disabilities can be present from birth or may be acquired.

ACTIVITY

Look at the following examples of disabled clients and decide what physical, intellectual, emotional and social needs they have. Discuss what may happen if these needs are not met.

1. Vikram is a 20-year-old student with cerebral palsy. He has normal intelligence but he has a problem with mobility and speech. He finds it difficult to walk long distances. He is following a full-time course at a local college. He finds it difficult to make friends.

2. Jessica is 3-years-old. She has Downs Syndrome. At the moment she is in a nursery class attached to a mainstream infants school. Jessica is very active and needs constant supervision. Her parents want her to go to the infants school, but the teachers feel her needs will be met more effectively in a Special School. Jessica's speech and writing skills are slow to develop, although she is able to use the toilet and feed herself. Other children in the class tend to avoid her.

3. Mark is 26. He had a car accident when he was 18. He is a wheelchair user. At the moment he works in the office of a charity for disabled people as a fundraiser. He wants to move to a flat and be independent. Mark has an adapted car. He can manage his own personal care, but needs help with housework and shopping.

4. Ted is 55. When he was 40 he travelled abroad for his company. He contracted a rare virus which left him paralysed from the neck down. He has regained some use in his arms and can feed himself, but he is dependent on others for his personal care and transport. He lives at home with his wife. The house has been adapted. He has to be careful to avoid coughs and colds, as these can have a serious effect on his lungs. He spends a lot of time advising other disabled people and being involved in several voluntary groups.

In this section we have looked at different client groups and identified their needs.

Some of these needs may be met by the family members or by the individual themselves. However, additional support may sometimes be needed from other health and social care workers.

If the needs of these people are not met, there may be serious problems.

Figure 2.7 shows the various workers that may be involved in the different client groups. We will look at the roles of these workers later in this chapter.

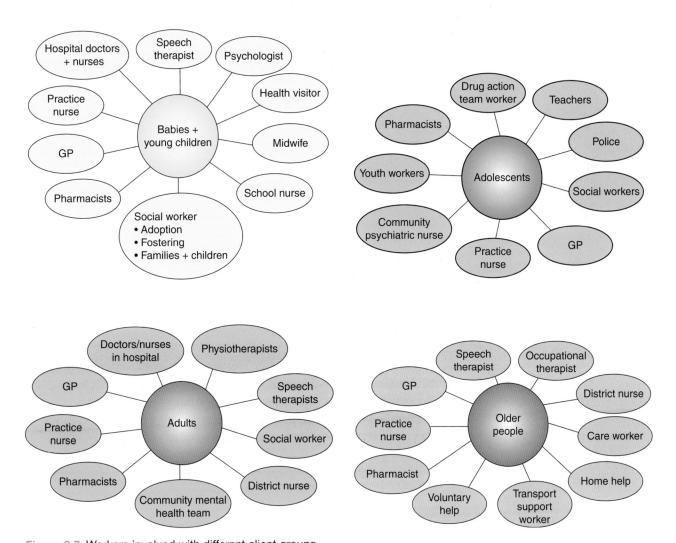

Figure 2.7 Workers involved with different client groups

How do health, social care and early years services respond to the needs and demands of the different groups?

Services for different groups respond in a variety of ways depending on the needs of the group or the individuals with in it. In all services a careful assessment is made of a person's needs. For example:

- a doctor may refer a child with a breathing problem to a paediatrician, who will assess the child and decide what treatment is suitable
- a worried family member may call a social worker because she is concerned about an 80-year old relative who can no longer cope at home. The social

worker may carry out an assessment of the older person's needs and decide if she requires a service to help her cope at home. The social care assessment will cover all aspects of the older person, including her financial position as clients contribute to social care in England.

- a young man may need emergency treatment after a serious accident. An ambulance may take him if it is not possible for him to make his own way to hospital. At the local hospital, in the A&E Unit, he will be assessed and, depending on his injury, may be treated and discharged home that day, or operated upon and admitted to a ward for further observation.

In all these examples you can see that the first approach to a client or patient to a service is for an assessment to be carried out and then the appropriate service to be offered. Services are developed partly as a result of changes in society – such as an increase in life expectancy – and partly because of economic and political pressures.

Universal services

Universal services are those that are available throughout the UK. These services include the National Health Service, Social Services and the Education Services. These are called statutory services because they have been set up as a result of legislation (laws) and they have to be available to everybody in every area of the UK.

Targeted services

Certain services are provided to certain groups in certain areas because they are seen to be needed. They may be targeted because of government policy or health improvement aims. Recent examples of these are 'stop smoking' clinics and obesity programmes that have been set up.

KEY TERM

Primary care trust (PCT) – a NHS organisation that covers a particular region and employs doctors, nurses and other staff. It also commissions (buys) services from hospitals and other services to treat patients.

EXAMPLE

In a South London primary care trust, research has found that one in five children starting primary schools is obese. After-school activity programmes have been set up; parents are given advice about what foods to give their children, and children who lose weight are offered rewards such as cinema tickets.

Meeting social policy goals

Social policy is about the government's plans to provide services in the following key areas:

- education
- housing
- income management (either through benefits or earned income)
- health services
- social services
- early years services.

Social policy is affected by certain factors (see Figure 2.8).

We will now look at one example of social policy where the government has tried to reduce child poverty in the UK.

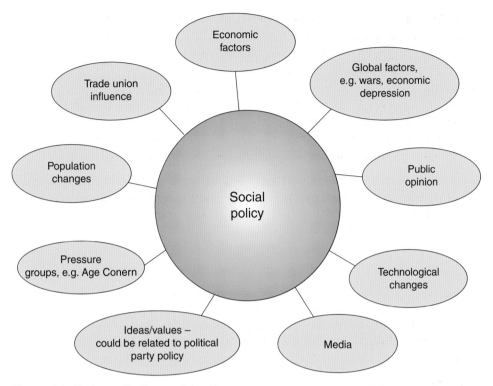

Figure 2.8 Factors affecting social policy

Poverty is difficult to define. Within the European Union, the poverty line is usually drawn at below 50% of the average income in that particular society. In the past, National Assistance (i.e. benefits paid by the State) was based on the minimum level of income required to sustain life. This amount was criticised as it meant that no one could do anything else but exist on this amount – no birthday cards or presents, no holidays and no social activity, including using transport, were possible. In the UK in 2008, poverty is defined as households that have an income below 60% of the average median income.

What is the government planning to do to reduce child poverty?

In 2007 the government set up a Child Poverty Unit. This new team is drawn from different sections of the government, such as the Department of Health (DOH), Department for Work and Pensions (DWP) and the Department for Children, Schools and Families (DCSF). The Child Poverty Unit aims to halve child poverty by 2010 and remove it completely by 2020.

In the last 20 years the proportion of children in low income households has doubled. In the UK, one in five low-income families had no one in work and one in every three children were living in poverty.

What will the government do?

- increase the income of families in poverty by encouraging parents back to work through education and training
- early years services and schools will support children from poorer families so that they do well both at school and in work as adults
- health and social care services will provide high-quality care for all families

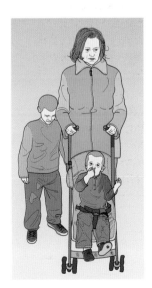

Figure 2.9 Child poverty is a serious issue in the UK

- benefits such as Child Tax Credits and Child Benefits will provide financial help to parents
- parents will be supported through children's centres, voluntary organisations and health care professionals.

Many children in poverty are in single parent families. This group will also be encouraged back to work with the government paying for child care costs. The Unit also wants to develop a child care workforce so that the standards of child care are good in all parts of the UK.

In addition the Unit is working to break the cycle of deprivation; this is where the children of parents in poverty are more likely to be in poverty themselves. This could be done through providing better housing for poor families, good meals in schools made available for all children and improving health and social care services for all children and families.

Reducing child poverty is not just about increasing the income that poor families receive but making it possible for them to work and take part fully in the community.

Child poverty is one example of social policy. Other social policy programmes include reducing homelessness and drug misuse and supporting children and young people who are in care. These programmes are being developed in a partnership between the statutory sector (the local council and the health service), the voluntary sector and the private sector. Partnership is one of the key approaches used in all aspects of social policy.

How do the health service and local authorities assess the care needs of their population?

Identifying needs

Different regions of the UK have different needs. The local primary care trusts identify the needs of their population and then develop services to meet those needs. At the same time, national priorities are identified in health and social care, and national programmes are also introduced.

Examples of local health programmes to meet local needs:

- sexual health clinics aimed at young people, and contraceptive advice and support are offered in an area that has a high teenage pregnancy rate
- diabetes support clinics are specifically provided for women from Asian backgrounds, who are more likely to have diabetes.

Some of these programmes may be part of national schemes.

Examples of national health programmes to meet national needs:

- stop smoking programmes that have been developed locally as part of the national programme to reduce the numbers of people smoking
- reducing obesity levels among the population, focusing on young children, patients with high blood pressure, diabetes and heart problems.

In all these programmes, statistics such as causes of death and incidence of disease are collected, and the health needs of the population identified and plans are made to improve health.

Each year the primary care trust for each area produces a report. This report identifies the needs of the area and the plans to meet those needs are outlined. The PCT may identify needs in a variety of ways, through questionnaires, public meetings, group meetings, and so on. This process is called a health needs assessment, and is usually led by the Public Health Unit of the PCT.

Figure 2.10 shows an example of profiling a community to identify needs.

The local council does a similar exercise to establish needs for housing, transport and social care needs. Many of these exercises focus on the needs of particular groups, such as older people, disabled groups and children.

A recent change in how local needs are assessed has been made by the PCT and the local council working together to do a Joint Strategic Needs Assessment. This assessment will result in a five-year strategic plan. This plan will identify local and national priorities in health and social care (including children's services) and state how the needs will be met within an agreed time scale.

Who uses health, social care and early years services and why may they need them?

At every age people may need health and social care services for a variety of reasons.

<table>
<tr><td>KEY TERMS</td></tr>
<tr><td>Morbidity rates – the rate of disease in a population.
Mortality rates – the death rate in a population.</td></tr>
</table>

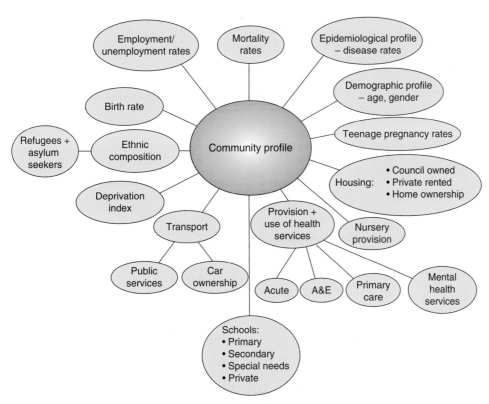

Figure 2.10 An example of profiling a community to identify needs

ACTIVITY

Discuss in your groups when you last attended a health or social care service? Why did you decide to go? Where did you decide to go?

Health and social care service providers are concerned that people should use the right service

ACTIVITY

Look at the following situations and decide where you might go for help.

1. You have had an upset stomach and you don't feel very well.
2. You fell off a ladder in the room you were decorating at home.
3. You are babysitting a neighbour's 2-year-old child, Ian. He looks and feels very hot; he has no energy and you are having trouble getting him to respond to you.
4. You came out of hospital after a car crash. You still ache a lot and the painkillers don't seem to be working.
5. You live next door to a young family. There always seems to be a lot of shouting and the two children look very thin and are dressed in summer clothes in the winter. They appear to wander round the street at all hours.
6. In your road there is an old lady – everyone calls her 'Batty Vera'. She wanders round the street and seems very confused about who she is and where she is.

One of the government's challenges is to encourage people to use the correct service if they don't feel well.

Look at Figure 2.11. This comes from an NHS leaflet.

Look again at the answers you gave. Would you change them now you have read the information about whom to see if you feel ill?

1. Many minor problems can be checked out with the pharmacist. Pharmacists are increasing their role in the community. Many pharmacists offer a range of free services such as advising you on your prescribed medicines and doing blood pressure checks.
2. The GP is available for routine and urgent cases and for patients who have been recently discharged from hospital.
3. You can take yourself to A & E (Accident and Emergency Services) if you feel you are in urgent need of treatment.
4. Dialling 999 should only be done in cases of real emergency – such as a suspected heart attack or in an accident.
5. Illnesses affecting young children and babies are quite frightening and in the case of Ian, urgent care is needed.
6. If you are worried about the safety of young children or older people you can phone social services. If you don't know what to do, there are various helplines and charities that can advise you. The NSPCC is always only a phone call away and they can discuss with you what may be the right thing to do.

KEY TERM

NSPCC – the National Society for the Prevention of Cruelty to Children.

In the UK most people are aware of those services that will give support 'from the cradle to the grave' and later in this chapter we will discuss how people access the service they require.

In the example we have discussed, most cases require short-term care. However, in the case of 'Batty Vera' her needs may increase and become permanent. Other examples of long-term care needs could include the following groups:

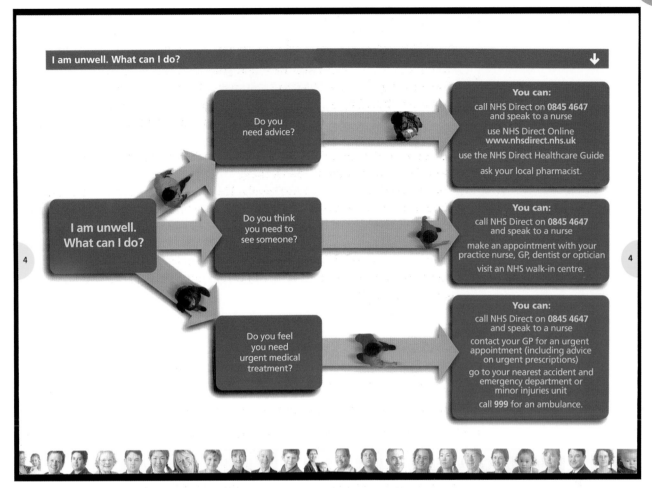

Figure 2.11 What to do if you feel ill

- people with specific needs such as disability
- older people who can no longer remain independent
- people who have severe mental health problems
- children who are born with disabilities such as cerebral palsy (CP).

How health care, social care and early years services are accessed

The range of services available to the different service users

In this section we will see that there are services to meet the needs of all age groups from infants to older people and including people with specific needs. There are four sectors of service provision (see Figure 2.12).

How have services developed and how are they organised ?

The basis of the NHS is that everyone should have access to free health care if they need it. NHS services try to provide services to everyone without discrimination on the basis of ethnicity, gender, social class, sexual orientation, where they live, or the illness they have. Both Social Services and the NHS services are statutory services and they have to conform to the Equality Legislation and also to the Human Rights Act in making sure that everyone is treated fairly.

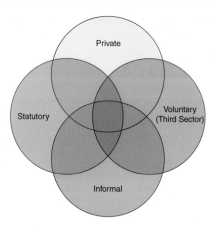

Figure 2.12 The four sectors of care

Social Services differ from the NHS, as many clients are means tested to see how much they should contribute to their care. Assessment of care needs is free, but the person may be charged for the service. When a person contacts social services because they think they need a service they will be screened; this means the social worker will decide if they have a need that should be met by social services. In order to make access to social services as fair as possible, there are national guidelines in place under the FACS system. FACS stands for Fair Access to Care Services and, after the assessment, social workers decide what level of need the client has. There are four levels of need which reflect the level of risk to the client. The lowest level of need is not seen as urgent; for example, someone needing help with shopping and housework. The highest level of need is at the level where the risk to the person is seen to be critical and the client will be assessed quickly and help provided. For example, if someone had dementia and was wandering around the streets at night time they could be at risk from falling or from attack. Remember Batty Vera? In social services, clients are assessed for their health and social care needs and they are also assessed financially through a means test.

Health and social care is organised differently in Wales, Scotland and Northern Ireland. Charging for health and social care in these regions differs, including the charge for prescriptions and for personal care.

Integrated children's services

Early years and children's services are also based on meeting the needs of children at risk. Child Protection policies safeguard children from risk. Some parents feel that certain groups still have problems in accessing services. Children with special needs are assessed through a Statement of Special Needs. In this Statement the support that is needed by the child is agreed with the parents, nurseries and schools. Schools have Special Educational Needs Co-ordinators (SENCOs) who are responsible for making sure that the child has enough support at school; this could be an assistant who stays with the child all the day, or for a few hours a week. Parents of special needs children often feel they have difficulty getting enough support for their child. In education there are problems of making sure all children have equal access to services such as schools and nurseries.

Many parents feel that their child can be supported more fully by trained staff in a special needs school. Government policy has supported the inclusion of children with special needs in mainstream schools so that they are included in society, rather than excluded by being in a special school.

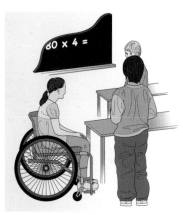

Figure 2.13 Integration into the mainstream school

Some towns which have a few popular schools that everyone wants to go to, have used a 'lottery system' so that everyone has an equal chance to go to the school of their choice when they go to secondary school.

DISCUSSION

Do you think children should be offered places in popular schools by a lottery system? What are the good things and bad things about doing that?

Do you think children with special needs should go to separate schools or should they be in mainstream schools?

Extended services

A recent example of extended services in education is the development of children's centres. These centres are open from 8 am to 6 pm and provide care for babies and young children.

Other examples of extended services can be walk-in centres that are usually open when GP surgeries are closed. GPs are being encouraged by the government to open surgeries and close later so that workers can make appointments during the extended hours.

Local authority services

Statutory social care

The government finances a range of statutory services through the local authorities. Money is spent by the local authority on local services such as:

- education, including early years services
- social services, for all age groups and client groups.

The local authority receives money from:

- central government
- payment for services, and
- the rates that are paid by the local community.

There are four main areas of social care provision:

1. Residential care – care provided in residential homes.
2. Domiciliary care – care provided in the client's own home.
3. Day care – care provided at special centres in the community.
4. Field work – care provided by social workers who care for particular client groups.

These are the groups that could require support:

- older people
- people with learning difficulties
- people with mental health problems
- people with drug and alcohol problems
- people with AIDS and HIV
- refugees
- homeless people.

Services provided by social services include the following:

- assessing needs
- providing personal help
- social work
- day care facilities
- residential and respite care facilities
- occupational therapy
- rehabilitation
- supplying specialist equipment
- an emergency service, 24 hours a day, 365 days a year.

Access to social care is through referral and assessment.

Figure 2.14 shows the social care services available for different client groups.

National policy is trying to achieve fairness across the country as, at the moment, some social service departments charge different rates for the same service. The government introduced the Fair Access to Care Services scheme, which assesses people according to their need for a service. However, local authorities have some choice in what services they deliver.

Examples of services that the social services have a duty to provide include:

- an initial assessment of need – this is a free service
- housing for people with mental health problems who have been discharged from hospital.

Examples of services that the social services may choose to provide include:

- home care facilities
- meals on wheels.

The social services provide some services directly, but nowadays they often buy these services from private or voluntary organisations.

Private provision in health care, social care and early years services

Private provision in health care can include private hospitals that treat patients as both in-patients and out-patients. Consultants also offer private appointments. Some treatment centres provide specific services such as cataract operations, hip and knee replacements and hernia operations. Patients may be treated at the centres and the operation paid for by the NHS, or patients will pay for the treatment themselves, either from savings, or through an insurance scheme.

Private provision in social care includes private residential and nursing homes, where the individual may pay the full cost of care. Social services and the NHS may pay, either part of the cost, or the whole cost.

Private provision in children's services includes private nurseries, adoption agencies, nannies and private nursery nurses.

Private companies

Because running a residential home, or providing private domiciliary or nursing care, can be quite expensive to set up and maintain, many private companies own a chain of residential homes or hospitals (such as BUPA). Nursing agencies, social care agencies and nannying agencies are all examples of private companies that provide care.

Self-employed practitioners

Many people are self-employed. Changes in the contract for dentists which changed the way dentists were paid for their work by the NHS, caused many

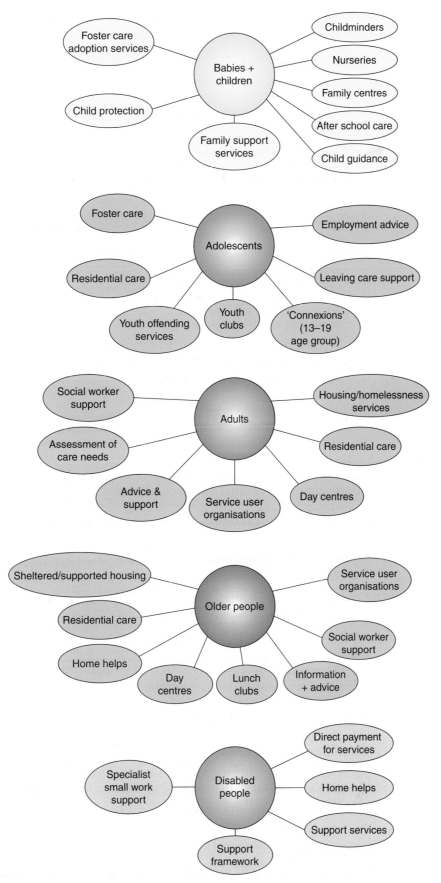

Figure 2.14 The social care services available for different client groups

dentists to leave the service and to set up as self-employed practitioners. Other groups of practitioners that are self-employed and work in the community include private physiotherapists, midwives and podiatrists. Alternative practitioners are another example of self-employed practitioners.

Alternative therapists

These are private services offered in the community. Therapies include:

- homeopathy
- osteopathy
- chiropractic
- acupuncture.

ACTIVITY

1. Use the local telephone directory or Yellow Pages to find the types of alternative therapist in your area. You can find out more about some alternative therapies on the following websites:
   www.acupuncture.org.uk
   www.homeopathyorg.uk/page/

2. In pairs, prepare a short talk to give to the rest of the class on an alternative therapy of your choice.

KEY TERMS

Direct care – services that are provided by practitioners to clients directly. For example, the GP who examines a patient; a nurse who changes a dressing; a midwife who delivers a baby; a nursery nurse who changes a nappy.

Indirect care – services that are provided by workers who support the direct care practitioner; for example, receptionists in a GP surgery; a cleaner who empties the bins; a porter who takes a mother to the delivery room in a wheelchair; a practice manager who organises the rotas of the receptionists.

Outsourcing of indirect care services

With the NHS Community Care Act (1990) NHS organisations were able to use other private providers for the services used in a hospital. Up until the Act, cleaners, caterers, and hospital security workers, including porters, had been directly employed by the hospital. Nowadays, most of these services are provided by private companies that have a contract with the hospital. If the hospital has several companies competing for the work, it may choose the company that is the cheapest. Can you think of any problems with this?

DISCUSSION

You may have thought that there could be problems of quality if the meals provided are cheaper. Many London hospitals use a catering company based in Wales. Food has to be transported a long way and is reheated in the hospital using the 'cook chill method'. If cleaning companies employ staff and pay them low wages, they may not be interested in the work and not do it properly. You may have seen news reports of poor standards of cleaning in hospitals.

Voluntary services or the Third Sector

Many voluntary organisations offer a range of services. As the role of the local council has changed from providing services to buying in services, the council may buy its services from a range of organisations.

Since the 1990 NHS and Community Care Act, voluntary organisations have become providers of a great deal of care.

Figure 2.15 shows some of the range of services that are provided by voluntary organisations in a London borough.

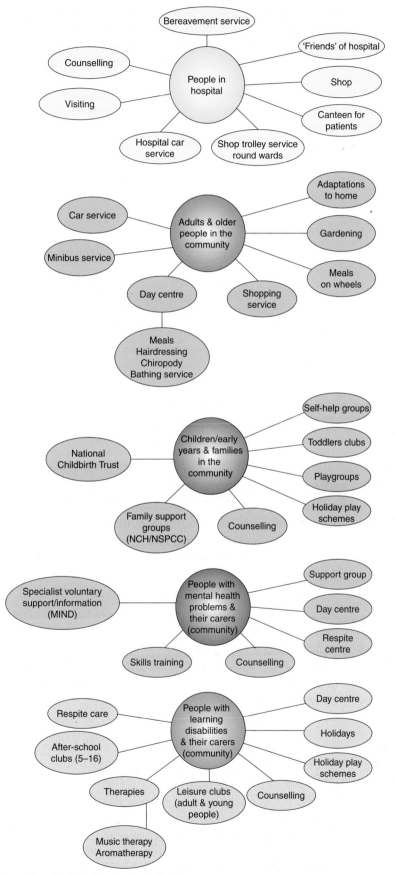

Figure 2.15 Services offered by the Third (voluntary) Sector

(Note: Although some services may be provided by volunteers, voluntary organisations also employ people to provide services.)

Figure 2.16 shows an example of the income received by a voluntary organisation.

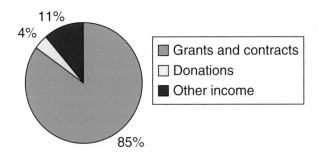

Figure 2.16 The income from a local voluntary organisation

ACTIVITY

Look at Figure 2.16 carefully. You can see that most of its income comes from grants and contracts from the statutory sector.

Many voluntary organisations started off as small local groups and then became national organisations. Volunteers are essential if local groups are going to be able to succeed.

ACTIVITY

Find out about a voluntary organisation in your area. All Third Sector organisations produce an annual report; this is a useful starting point for your research. Most organisations have a website nowadays. Find out which groups of people the organisation assists. Does it provide services or does it act as a pressure group to improve services?

For example, the Alzheimer's Society is a national organisation, but it has local branches which provide services to clients with Alzheimer's disease. With the recent controversy over the drugs that are available to people suffering with Alzheimer's, many branches became involved in marches, demonstrations and interviews for the press, in order to raise awareness of issues that affect this group of people.

Charities

The definition of a charity is a body or trust that is for a charitable purpose and is for the public benefit.

Most voluntary organisations are registered charities. Charities are regulated by the Charity Commission. Charities have to publish annual accounts and these are available on the Charity Commission's website.

See www.charity-commission.gov.uk.

Local support groups

Many local support groups develop in response to a need that is felt by a group of people in a particular area. Examples of support groups can be church or faith-based groups; groups that support mothers or informal carers; groups that give support to people who have a particular disease or illness.

Not-for-profit organisations

Voluntary organisations do not have shareholders. They provide services for people in their community usually paid for (or commissioned) by health and social care organisations. Any surplus money is put back into the organisation to develop services still further.

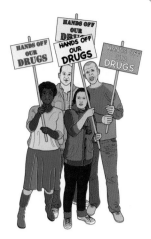

Figure 2.17 People demonstrating about the withdrawal of drugs from Alzheimer's patients

Informal provision

Informal provision of health, social care and early years services can be offered in the community by different groups, such as:

- churches
- mother and baby clubs
- babysitting circles
- volunteer sitters for older neighbours to keep them company
- volunteer drivers who take people to hospital, to doctors appointments.

Family and friends offer informal support to individuals. Grandparents offer a lot of informal childcare. Neighbours used to be a source of informal support, but recent research shows that many people no longer know their neighbours!

Carers

There are six million carers in the UK, but who are they?

A carer is anyone who is helping to look after a partner, friend or relative who, because of illness, old age or disability may not be able to manage at home without help.

Carers save the government an estimated £67 billion every year by caring for people at home. Without this informal care, many people would have to live in residential care.

It has been estimated that there are 900,000 people who care for someone for more than 50 hours each week.

Many people who are carers find that caring is very tiring, and this affects the paid work they do. They become stressed and may have to move from full-time work to part-time work, or give up work altogether.

Caring can be very time-consuming. The Princess Royal Trust for Carers found that 58% of carers aged 16+ spend more than 15 hours a day caring. If there are only 24 hours in a day, this doesn't leave much time for doing other things.

What does caring involve?

Caring could be:

- helping someone to get up in the morning and go to bed at night
- cooking a meal and helping the person eat it
- helping someone have a bath and use the toilet.

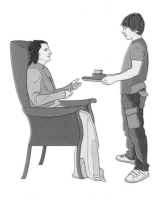

Figure 2.18 A young carer

Young carers

Recent research shows that there may be many young carers under the age of 16. What do you think is the age of the youngest carer: 14, 12, 10, 8, or 6?

The youngest carer found by a carers' centre was 6-years-old.

Young carers who are primary carers are more likely to care for someone with a physical disability (32%) or a mental health problem (21%).

Support for young carers

Thirty-three per cent of the young carers interviewed in a research project said that their teachers did not know they were looking after someone. Many young carers do not tell their friends that they are carers, as they feel they would be laughed at and no one would want to be friends with them. They try to keep their caring role a secret.

Research shows that 79% of young female carers have been bullied at school, and that 60% of young male carers have also experienced bullying. These young people suffered verbal, physical and emotional abuse, and many truanted from school as a result.

Is there a carers' centre near you? If there is, find out what services it offers.

Figure 2.19 shows the services offered by a centre in South London.

In this section we have seen how a range of providers offer services to different clients.

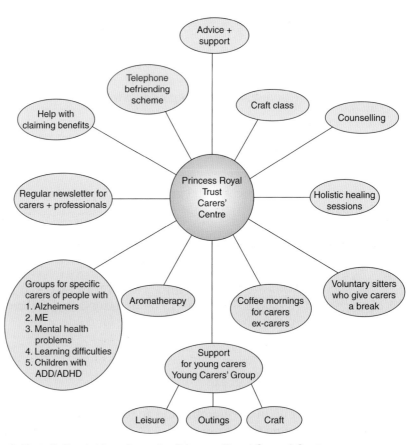

Figure 2.19 Activities taking place at a Princess Royal Carers' Centre

National organisation of health, social care and early years services

The national organisation of the NHS.

The Department of Health is the national government department in charge of the organisation of the Health Service in the UK. Wales, Scotland and Ireland control the organisation of health and social care in their regions.

The Secretary of State for Health has overall responsibility for the NHS.

Do you know his/her name?

In England there are 10 Strategic Health Authorities which oversee the delivery of health services by the hospital trusts, mental health trusts and primary care trusts.

There are 152 PCTs in England, which plan and deliver services.

They must:

- assess the health needs of the population
- draw up a plan to meet those needs, working in partnership with the local authority and the voluntary sector.

Primary care trusts employ staff and offer services. PCTs buy services from the acute hospitals and the mental health trusts. These three trusts work together with the local authority and the Third Sector to provide services for the local population.

All Trusts and health authorities have to produce annual reports, and these could give you useful information for your projects.

Figure 2.20 shows the different health services available for different client groups.

> ### KEY TERMS
>
> **Primary care** – health care that takes place in the community and is given by the Primary Health Care Team – the GP, practice nurses, health visitors, district nurses, dentists, pharmacists, and opticians.
>
> **Secondary care** – is care that is given in hospitals.
>
> **Tertiary care** – is care that is given in specialist hospitals – for example cancer hospitals.

NHS Trusts

NHS Hospital Trusts

Under the 1990 NHS and Community Care Act, hospitals became self-governing trusts. This meant they were able to do the following:

- buy, own and sell land and services
- develop their own management systems
- employ their own staff and set out their own terms and conditions of employment (they also used outside companies for cleaning and catering services)
- raise money through developing private patient services, renting out shops in the hospital, car park charges and other ways of raising income.

Hospital trusts have to produce an annual report, which provides statistics on numbers of patients treated, length of waiting lists, as well as planned developments.

It may be useful if you look at a copy of a hospital trust report. They should be in your local library, or else you can obtain one directly from the hospital. They are usually accessible on the Trust website

Mental Health Trusts

Because of the specialist care needed for people with mental health problems, mental health trusts have been developed that link hospital and community care

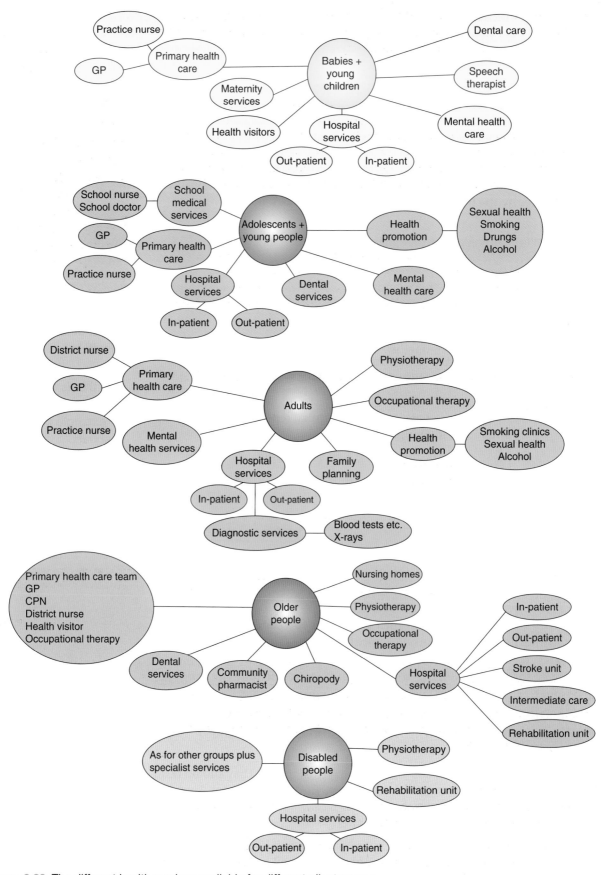

Figure 2.20 The different health services available for different client groups

for their patients. Community psychiatric nurses are part of the outreach team that provides services such as day centres and drop-in centres for patients, as well as providing a 24-hour service in the community.

Foundation Trusts

In 2006 there were 52 NHS Foundation Trusts. Foundations Trusts still offer NHS services but they are free-standing organisations. This means they are not under the control of the Health Secretary. They can invest in developing new services. Patients and staff can become members of Foundation Trusts and they elect a Board of Governors, so they are involved in the decision making that takes place. It is expected that all mental health trusts and hospital trusts will become Foundation Trusts in the next few years

Day surgery

Because of changes in technology, many hospitals offer day surgery for routine operations such as the removal of wisdom teeth, the removal of cataracts and other minor operations that require a general anaesthetic. More GPs are offering minor surgery in their practices. This means that the number of beds needed in hospitals has gone down.

Emergency services

NHS hospitals provide emergency services 24 hours a day. On entry to A & E (accident and emergency), you will be seen immediately by a triage nurse who will assess your need for treatment.

NHS Direct

This is a 24-hour helpline staffed by nurses who will give advice on the telephone. It covers England and Wales.

Nurses on NHS Direct can advise callers to self-care, to see the pharmacist or to see their GP. They can also advise callers to dial 999 or to attend A & E.

NHS walk-in centres

These centres are being developed in major towns and cities. They are open from 7 am to 10 pm for advice and clinical treatment by nurses and doctors. As the name suggests, you can walk in without an appointment.

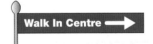

Figure 2.21 Walk in centres

NHS Internet service

The website, www.nhsdirect.nhs.uk was launched in December 1999. This website gives information about the NHS and how to use it. It also includes pages on diseases and their treatment. It is an interactive website that allows users to describe their symptoms and to self-diagnose (which could cause problems!). Depending on your answers, the user will be advised to self-care, see the GP or pharmacist, or phone NHS Direct or 999.

The National Organisation of Social Care

Since devolution, Scotland, Wales and Northern Ireland have their own systems of care. In this section we will focus on care in England.

The Secretary of State for Health has overall responsibility for the national organisation of both Health and Social care services. Social Services departments control the social services in each local authority and the Director of Social

---

KEY TERM

Triage nurse – a trained nurse who assesses your needs when you arrive at A & E.

It is hoped that the use of A & E for minor problems will be reduced, and that people will contact NHS Direct and will either self-care, see their GP or consult a pharmacist.

Service is in charge of the Social Services Department. The powers of Local Authorities are decided by Parliament. Statutory services are those that *have* to be provided, but each local social services department can decide on what additional services they may provide and the charges that will be made for these services.

The government finances a range of statutory services through the local authorities. Money is spent by the local authority on local services including:

- education – including early years services
- social services – for all age groups and client groups.

The local authority receives money from central government, from payment for services and also from the rates that are paid by the local community.

The services provided and the client groups that are supported by social services are outlined on page 82.

The national organisation of early years services

There is an overlap in services provided for the health care, social care and education services provided for children.

Primary health care

Most of the care of young children is undertaken by parents. With less time spent in hospital, children are more likely to be looked after in their own homes. GPs have responsibility for all the children in their practice. Preventative services such as routine immunisations, developmental checks and advising parents are all part of the work of the Primary Health Care Team (PHCT).

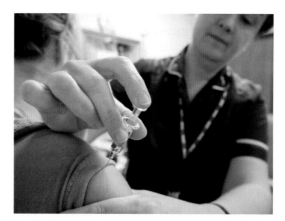

Figure 2.22 Immunisations are an important part of caring for young children

School services

The government's Healthier Schools Programme means healthier children. School nurses promote the health of the children and give help and advice to parents and pupils.

Each school has a named nurse who visits the school regularly and refers children to other services in the community.

There are also paediatric nurses employed by the hospital or PCTs, who visit children in their own homes to continue treatment, or to offer support after a stay in hospital. The duties of a community paediatric nurse can include the following:

- follow-up care after treatment in A & E
- post-operative care
- removal of stitches, dressing of wounds, giving injections
- advising and training parents in giving care.

Emergency health services for children

Apart from the out-of-hours service offered by GPs, and general hospitals who have a children's department, there are specialist children's hospitals that look after children until the age of 16. The hospitals are organised so that children feel comfortable. Often the departments and wards are brightly painted with pictures and other decorations.

Secondary health services for early years

Secondary care is provided in hospitals. Hospital pediatricians provide emergency and routine surgery for children. GPs will refer children to outpatient departments, where they can be seen by the specialist team. Nowadays, parents are encouraged to stay with their children in hospital, and overnight accommodation is offered to them.

Social Services Early Years

Children's Services

The Children Act of 2004 required local councils to set up Local Safeguarding Boards, which would include workers from all the services that provide children services. Local councils also had to appoint a Director of Children's Services who would lead a separate department.

The local social service departments provide a range of services for young children. These services may be provided directly by social services, or they are provided in partnership with the Third Sector, or they are purchased from private or other independent sector providers.

Statutory provision of children's services

The Children Act (1989) was an important piece of legislation that stated '*the services that must be provided for those children assessed as being in need*':

- day care for children under five and not at school
- care and supervised activities outside school hours and during school holidays
- accommodation if required, if children are lost, abandoned or without a carer that can provide accommodation.

Social Services must also provide:

- assessment of needs
- an emergency service 24 hours a day, 365 days a year.

Social services may also provide the following caring services for children and their families:

- occupational therapy
- supplying specialist equipment
- respite care
- personal help.

The organisation of a children's social services department

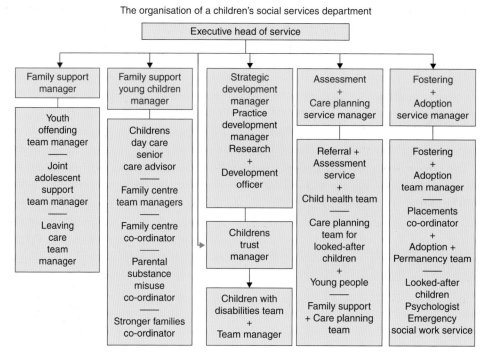

Figure 2.23 A Chidren's Department

Day care services and childminders

Day care service providers and childminders must be registered with Ofsted.

Fostering and adoption

The Children Act (1989) states that the local authority must make arrangements to enable the child to live with their family unless this would harm the child. Foster carers are approved by either the local authority, or by a voluntary or private organisation. Local authorities have to keep a register of foster carers in the area and keep records of children placed with them.

The law related to adoption is complicated (Adoption Act 1979 and Children Act 1989). An adoption order transfers all the responsibilities of the parent to the adopters. An adopter has to be:

- at least 21
- resident in the UK
- able to meet the criteria of the relevant adoption agency or local authority.

Non-statutory provision

Examples of non-statutory provision in the community would include:

- private nurseries
- private residential homes
- private fostering and adoption agencies.

These are privately run as a business, but the services are used and paid for by the social services.

Independent voluntary provision for early years can include:

- toddlers' clubs
- care for children with special needs (Mencap services)

- holiday care
- mother and child support groups.

Figure 2.24 is an example of a voluntary service for families with young children.

Family Focus is a registered charity that was set up to protect and preserve the mental and physical health of families with children under the age of five.

Family Focus aims to:

- work alongside parents to develop family life skills
- help parents enjoy parenthood
- help parents to cope with the daily pressures of life.

To do this, parents can take part in a parenting skills course that includes:

- child development
- managing behaviour
- meeting needs of children and parents
- the importance of play.

There are also charities involved with the protection of young children. The most well-known of these is the NSPCC (National Society for the Prevention of Cruelty to Children). The NSPCC advises parents on child care, supports families who are finding it difficult to cope with their children, as well as investigating cases of abuse and cruelty to children.

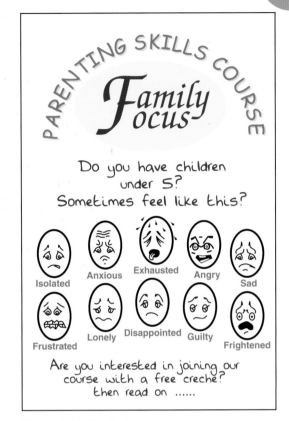

Figure 2.24 Family Focus

Informal provision

Much of the care of young children is arranged on an informal basis. For example, friends and neighbours may do unpaid babysitting; local churches may run mother and toddler clubs.

Informal care for all client groups

The focus for care has moved away from long-stay hospitals into the community. Although the Primary Health Care Team offers health care in the community, family, friends and neighbours offer more and more informal care. Under the 1990 NHS Community Care Act, long-stay hospitals were closed and patients moved into the community. People with learning disabilities, physical disabilities and mental health problems are now cared for in the community, and in practice this means by the family.

In this section we have seen how a range of providers offer services to different clients.

ACTIVITY

Look at the following list and decide whether each service is statutory, voluntary, private or informal.

1. A married daughter looking after her 75-year-old mother
2. A GP (general practitioner or family doctor)

(continued)

ACTIVITY – (continued)

3. A 'Meals on Wheels' service
4. A consultant working in a private hospital

Did you manage to identify all the service providers and decide whether they were, statutory, voluntary, private or informal?

You could make up your own case studies of clients from the different groups – babies and children, adolescents, adults and disabled people, and decide what services they may use and who would provide them.

Partnership working and multi-agency working

Nowadays, more and more partnership working is taking place in health and social care services.

Sure Start children's centres

These centres have been developed under the Ten Year Child Care Strategy started by the government. These centres were set up to support children who were living in areas of deprivation. Multi-disciplinary teams work at the centre, so they can support mothers and their children from pregnancy to school age.

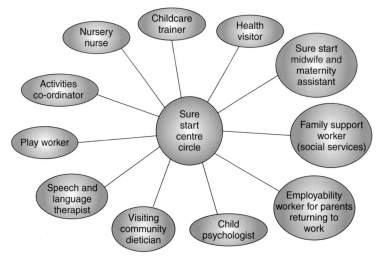

Multy-disciplinary team at a Sure Start centre

Figure 2.25 A multi-disciplinary team at a Sure Start centre

KEY TERMS

Partnership working – when two or more organisations work together- for example the local health trust and social services providing a podiatry service.

Podiatry sometimes known as **chiropody** – a service provided by a trained professional who cares for the feet, including minor surgery.

KEY TERM

Multi-disciplinary team – a team of professionals working together; this could be health visitors, district nurse and social workers.

Virtual wards

In 2006 certain PCTs developed 'virtual wards'. People are looked after in their own beds at home so there is no real ward, but the organisation of health care workers reflects what happens in a hospital ward. Each virtual ward can care for 100 patients. These patients are those who are regular attenders at A & E and frequently admitted to hospital. Each ward has the following staff:

- a community matron
- nurses
- a health visitor
- a pharmacist
- a social worker
- a physiotherapist
- a volunteer helper
- a ward clerk.

There is a link with local mental health services. Specialist staff also visit several 'virtual wards' in the area. For example, specialist practitioners in asthma, heart failure, continence, drug and alcohol service, dietitian.

Communication between professionals is by regular emails giving up-to-date reports on the patients. When patients improve they are discharged from the 'virtual ward', in the same way as if they were in hospital, and a discharge letter is sent to the GP practice and to the patient.

This new model of care is seen to have many advantages, especially for older people who are in and out of hospital and prefer to be at home with proper support. It is likely that there will be more 'virtual wards' in the future.

Case Study A multi-agency disability team

In 2007 a PCT in Greater London reviewed the day hospitals that were providing services for people with disabilities following falls, strokes and other problems. The new service was called OPARS (The Older Peoples Assessment and Rehabilitation Service). People who need the services are referred by their GP. At the centre, people are assessed by the multi-agency team. This team includes doctors, nurses, a physiotherapist, and an occupational therapist. Social services and voluntary groups are also involved at the centre as it is an opportunity for patients to receive information about services in the area and the benefits they may be entitled to. It is called a multi-agency team as the workers come from different health and social care organisations.

Local authority extended services provision

We have already seen the example of an extended school as an example of local authority provision. However, there is also a duty social worker who is responsible for all emergency cases out of working hours and on holidays and weekends.

How health, social care and early years services are provided

The ways in which service users access health, social care and early years services are accessed

Methods of referral

The ways that people gain access to care services are known as methods of referral. You should know about the different methods that exist.

Self-referral

This is when people decide to go and ask for the services themselves. Examples of self-referral are:

- going to the local A & E department when you have an accident
- making an appointment to see the GP

> **KEY TERM**
>
> **Multi-agency teams** – are those that have staff that could be employed by the local hospital trust or PCT, as well as therapists employed by social services and volunteers from the Third Sector.

Key worker – now usually called the lead professional

Whenever a patient or client attends hospital or is involved with a multi-disciplinary team in the community, they are given the name of the professional who is the person to contact if they have any queries. In hospital this would be a named nurse; in the community it could be a nurse, a social worker or a therapist (e.g. a physiotherapist). The reason one person is nominated as the key professional is that there is no confusion about who to contact when any queries arise.

- going to a genito-urinary medical (GUM) clinic for treatment of sexually transmitted diseases
- contacting the health visitor or practice nurse for advice or an appointment.

Self-referral is developing as the health and care services change. In the NHS, walk-in centres have been developed, where people can go for advice and treatment. The use of the phone service NHS Direct is another example.

Many of the new services on offer are a way of encouraging people to self-refer to appropriate services. Accident and Emergency services often find they are caring for people who could use other services, including the pharmacist. This could mean that serious emergencies may not get the prompt help they need.

All GP surgeries are required to produce a booklet giving information to patients about how to treat common conditions. See if you can find this at your local surgery.

Professional referral

This means that the person will be referred by the doctor, nurse, teacher or social worker to see a specialist or other professional. Examples of this would include:

- the GP making an appointment for a patient to see a consultant in the out-patient department of a hospital
- the psychiatrist referring a patient to a CPN (community psychiatric nurse)
- a teacher referring a disruptive pupil to the educational psychologist
- a health visitor referring a patient to the social work team.

Referrals to hospital for appointments can take a long time, and there are various government initiatives to reduce waiting lists for out-patient appointments. These include:

- encouraging the use of specialist GPs who will undertake procedures, usually done in hospital
- using outreach clinics, where the consultant visits a local health centre and sees patients near their own home
- changing arrangements for making appointments so that patients can choose a date and time convenient for them.

Third-party referral

There are a number of examples of third-party referral, which is when a person is put in contact with a service by a friend, relative or neighbour who is not employed as a care practitioner. Voluntary services – such as Age Concern – are often accessed by people who have heard about them from a friend. There are various voluntary groups that give advice about services. Many people do not use services that are available because they are not aware of their existence.

In some areas, there are information packs giving information about services available. These are often placed in libraries or health centres. Sometimes the people who need the information do not attend these places.

ACTIVITY

Can you think of other ways to inform people of services? Not everyone has the Internet, and we will see in the next section that there are all kinds of barriers to accessing care services.

Barriers to accessing services

Physical barriers

Many older GP practices have stairs, either to the front door or to the consulting rooms, which can make it difficult for people who have mobility problems, or for mothers using prams and pushchairs.

Under the Disability Discrimination legislation (2004), public services should make arrangements for disabled people; this could include the development of lifts in railways stations and disabled toilets in public buildings. However, the legislation only says that reasonable adjustments could be made, so a dental surgery may say they cannot afford to move the treatment room downstairs and they would refer the patient to a dentist who provides better access. By using the word 'reasonable', there is room for people to decide what is reasonable.

ACTIVITY

It may be a useful exercise to do a survey of public venues in your local high street and see what the access is like for disabled people. This would include shops, bars, pubs as well as GP clinics. Don't forget that disabled people are not just wheelchair users but may have sensory problems.

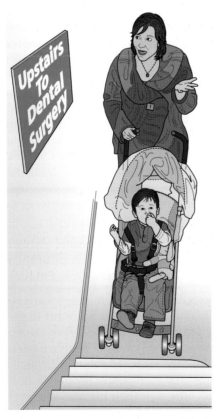

Figure 2.26 Access to health and care services can be difficult

People with sensory problems may also have difficulties of access. Phoning up to make an appointment can be a problem if you are deaf. Finding your way round a hospital can be difficult if you are visually impaired.

Psychological barriers

Men are less likely to make appointments to see the doctor because they feel it is 'unmanly'. As a result, many male patients finally see a doctor when the problem has become serious. Men are less likely than women to see their doctor if they are suffering from depression. Young men feel embarrassed seeing the doctor, especially about problems related to their genitals.

This is a particular concern, as there has been an increase in testicular cancer among young men. How could they be encouraged to see the doctor? There have been health programmes in secondary schools about testicular cancer and encouraging young men to examine themselves, but the results have been disappointing.

Certain services have a stigma attached to them, such as services treating sexually transmitted infections (STIs) and mental health services – which mean that people with these problems are unwilling to seek help for them.

Other psychological barriers can be phobias, when people develop an intense fear of, for example, needles (so they don't have injections) or of dental treatment.

Some phobias can be successfully treated, but the key to overcoming many of these barriers is through effective communication with patients, so that they understand why certain services may help them.

Some older people do not want strangers coming into their homes to look after them, or do not want to lose their independence.

Financial barriers

When the health service was set up in 1948, health care was to be free at the point of delivery. This included eye tests, prescriptions for medicines and dental treatment to certain groups. In 2008, many people are unwilling to use some of the services because of the cost involved. At the moment, a prescription costs £7.20 per item in England, although some groups are exempt. Another aspect of financial barriers to access, relates to dental treatment and eye tests. With certain exceptions, these have to be paid for in full, or else a contribution made towards the cost. Health workers fear that because of these charges, dental health will decline and serious eye conditions may not be detected. Refugees and asylum seekers are another group that experience problems of access to services for financial reasons.

The NHS (HC 12) produces a leaflet giving information about help with costs. Try to get hold of a copy at the post office or surgery. It might save you or your family some money!

Many social care services are now means tested and many people (especially older people) do not want to give information of a personal nature to the social worker. Depending upon the level of income and savings, older people have to contribute towards the costs of care, either in their own home or in residential care. This means that many older people do not receive the services they need, although their income and level of savings may mean that they would contribute little, if anything, towards their care. The financial assessment covers many pages of form filling, which can be difficult to do.

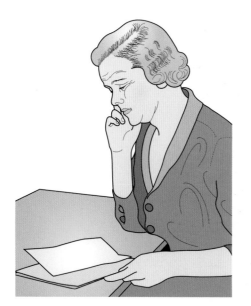

Figure 2.27 Filling in forms can be a problem

Geographical barriers

The different areas in Britain are very varied, with some densely populated towns and cities, and some rural areas that have limited facilities.

In some rural areas, local bus and train services have been reduced and there are problems for specialists in reaching outlying areas, as well as for patients accessing services. This problem is likely to increase with the proposed changes in the NHS, which mean that in the future there will be a concentration of specialist services in a few areas.

How might these concerns be addressed?

Help with travelling costs can be obtained through the NHS (see HC 12) but, again, the process is time-consuming. What provision might the hospital be able to offer? Sometimes there are volunteers who will drive people to appointments. We have to remember that all hospital trusts have to keep to a tight budget, so if money is spent on one area this reduces the money available for other services.

Cultural barriers

In some cultures women do not want to be cared for by a man. This has caused problems in the past, when Bangladeshi pregnant women did not attend antenatal clinics because they did not want to be examined by a man. This meant that difficulties with the baby were not recognised at an early stage. Nowadays, clinic nurses are more aware of these cultural differences and a female practitioner is usually available. Cultural differences include diet, religion and personal care, as well as the appropriate way to care for someone who has died. Nowadays, nurses and care workers are more aware of the importance of treating patients and clients according to their cultural beliefs.

Language barriers

In a study conducted in one London borough, it was found that the greatest problem facing refugees and asylum seekers was the lack of adequate interpreting services.

Some telephone interpreting services have been set up in GP practices in areas where there are people from other countries. These are helpful, but in many cases the use of a face-to-face interpreter is needed, especially when dealing with a complicated situation or when a family is involved in the discussion.

Receptionists in GP practices have found problems in identifying the language required. One way to solve this is through the use of a leaflet in which many languages are identified. Once the patient points to their language, the telephone interpreting service is contacted and the doctor conducts the consultation with the patient using the service. For complicated consultations that are booked in advance, it is possible to arrange for an interpreter to be present.

Some receptionists say that there have been cases where a young child in the family acts as interpreter for older family members. You can see the problem that this could cause.

Language barriers can also include deaf people who use signing to communicate. Signing is their first language, and they may have difficulty lip reading. In some services, it is now possible to book a signer to attend an appointment, or the person brings their own signer.

Many of the issues related to barriers of access could be resolved if the service provider was aware of the particular needs of the client before they attend for an appointment.

Resource barriers

This is a key issue in health and social care services. Local services are dependent on national funding from central government. All services need to show that they are able to work within a budget, and provide 'best value'. This means cost-effective services. Social services have to gain 7% of their income from charges they make to client groups. At the end of the financial year, budgets have to balance. A hospital trust cannot ask for more money if it overspends. It either has to carry the loss forward into the next year, or it has to cut services in order to stay within budget. Therefore, a ward may close or non-essential surgery may be cancelled.

Another key resource in health and care services is staff. At the moment there is a severe shortage of dentists, nurses and other staff in the NHS and in social care. One solution has been to recruit nurses from overseas, but this has its own problems.

Postcode lottery

PCTs are responsible for the prescribing budget in their area.

They decide which drugs will be paid for and which will not be supported. Some drugs are very expensive and may have limited value. This can mean that different parts of the country may have different policies on paying for expensive drugs. One way of reducing this unfairness has been with the development of the National Institute for Clinical Excellence (NICE). The role of NICE is to research new or expensive drugs and provide guidance as to whether the drug should be available on the NHS or not. NICE is also developing

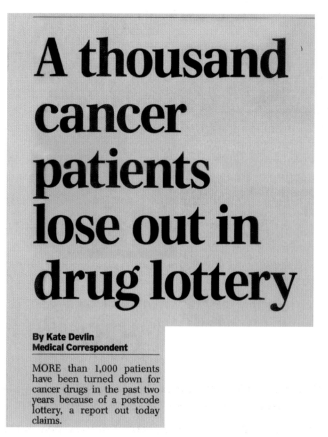

A thousand cancer patients lose out in drug lottery

By Kate Devlin
Medical Correspondent

MORE than 1,000 patients have been turned down for cancer drugs in the past two years because of a postcode lottery, a report out today claims.

Figure 2.28 Post code lottery

guidelines on referrals to hospital for conditions such as arthritis and skin complaints. It is hoped that by using national guidelines all patients will be treated fairly wherever they live in the UK.

Demand pressures

As more services develop, more people use them. One of the government's aims is to identify and support unpaid carers. At the moment many unpaid carers are unknown, but once they are identified and offered support this will put additional pressure on services in respite care for those cared for, as well as support services for the carers.

The increase in life expectancy means that the demand for services for older people has increased. One way of dealing with this is to encourage people to remain independent in their own homes, rather than use residential care or hospital services. However, staff are still needed to provide these services.

Increased demand for hip replacements in older people has led to government initiatives to speed up the process. Hip fractures are a common cause of hospital admission among older people. Prevention of accidents through exercise classes and safety checks in the home are additional programmes that have been developed.

Local demand on services will reflect the local population. For example, if the local population has a high number of children or older people, this will be reflected in the services needed.

Rationing of services

Newspaper articles have identified the problems of inequality of access to services, including the prescribing of drugs. Different local authorities may have different priorities in offering certain services. Some services are offered at the discretion of the local authority, and the charges made for care services can vary across the UK. At the moment, in Scotland all people aged 65 or over who are assessed by the social work department as needing care are entitled to a Free Personal Care Allowance of £147 a week. Anyone of any age who is in residential care in Scotland is also entitled to a Nursing Care Allowance of £67 a week. The cost of care above these amounts is means tested, but in England this would be charged for.

DISCUSSION

Think about how these barriers could be removed so that everyone can have equal access to the care they need.

The main work roles and skills of people who provide health, social care and early years services

What does care work involve and what skills do care practitioners need to perform their work roles?

Within the health and social care sectors, those staff who deliver care directly are called direct carers and those whose work is more indirectly involved with care are called indirect carers.

Examples of direct carers include: nurse, doctor, social worker, care assistant, nursery nurse.

Examples of indirect carers include: clinic clerk, receptionist, cleaner.

ACTIVITY

Look at the following list of examples of jobs and decide whether they are direct carers or indirect carers:

- hospital porter
- health visitor
- practice manager
- practice nurse
- chiropodist/podiatrist.

People who work as health workers usually look after patients who have health-related problems or conditions. People who work in social care are usually dealing with clients who have a range of personal and social needs.

ACTIVITY

Look at the following list of jobs and decide which are health care jobs and which are social care jobs:

- health visitor
- district nurse
- dentist
- pharmacist
- social worker
- care assistant
- housing officer.

KEY TERM

CACHE – stands for Council for the Awards in Childcare and Education

Direct carers in health and social care

Within each of these groups, there tends to be a common core of training followed by specialist training. For example, all doctors follow a standard medical training and those who choose to specialise in general practice complete additional training. Hospital play specialists have usually completed their initial training in childcare followed by a specialist course before they complete the hospital play specialist course.

Table 2.3 shows a list of qualities that a group of health and care workers identified as being essential for people working in health and social care. As you can see, personality traits and skills are listed, but the group also felt that these needed to be supported by knowledge. As a health or care worker you need to know why you do certain things.

Which 10 qualities would be most important in the role of the GP?

Personal Qualities	Skills
Sense of humour	Good communication skills:
Patient	- verbal
Tactful	- written
Sympathetic	- non-verbal
Respect for others	Legible writing
Caring	Professional approach
Reliable	Observation skills
Punctual	Assessment skills

Table 2.3 Essential qualities for people working in health and social care

Personal Qualities	Skills
Good health	Listening skills
Flexible approach	Supervision of others
Polite	Record keeping
Willing to learn	IT skills
Shows initiative	Numeracy skills
Confident	Can work as part of a team
Can work under pressure	Can work independently
Friendly	Able to drive a car
Respects confidentiality	Good manual dexterity
Smart appearance	Telephone skills
Attention to hygiene	Attention to health and safety
Understanding of others	
Gets on with everyone	

Table 2.3 (continued)

Underpinned by Knowledge

Although skills and personal qualities are important many jobs in health and social care require certain qualifications.

Job Title	Qualifications and training needed	Job role
Doctor	6 years medical training followed by additional training in specialist area – GP, surgery or medicine	Working in a hospital or community as a GP. Can work in a range of specialist hospitals
Registered Nurse (RN) – children – adult – mental health – learning disability	Different qualifications, diploma or degree. Requirements set by each institution. Mature students considered	Depends on the nature of the post. Could be specialist in stroke care, theatre work or district nursing
Community nurses	Registered Nurse Training qualification followed by specialist training	Range of posts – district nursing, health visiting, practice nursing, school nursing
Health visitors	Registered Nurse Training followed by specialist training	Working with families with children from birth to school age, advising pregnant women, and running a range of services including service for people suffering from incontinence. Giving general health advice
Midwives	Registered Nurse Training plus midwifery training or direct entry into midwifery training	Working with women during pregnancy, labour and delivery and post delivery. May work in hospital and in the community
Health care assistants (HCAs)	No minimum requirements needed. Initial training given plus NVQs	Personal care in hospital or community. Supporting qualified nurse and therapists
Portage workers	Experience of working with children under 5-years-of-age with a relevant qualification such as teaching, nursery nursing, nursing or social work plus training from the National Portage Association (NCA)	Working with children who have special needs or other development difficulties in schools or in their home. Developing programmes of activities to help their development, in partnership with the family

Table 2.4 Some direct carers in health and the qualifications they need for their work

Job Title	Qualifications and training needed	Job role
Child development workers	This covers a range of direct care workers, such as nursery nurses, portage workers, play specialists and child psychologists, so they will have a range of experience and qualifications such as CACHE, NVQ Level 2; Child Care or Degree in Psychology or Teacher Training Qualification	Working in hospital, children's centres and schools developing programmes to maximise the development of each child, according to their abilities. May work with children with special needs, physical or sensory disabilities or mental health problems
Early years practitioners	This term covers teachers, nursery teachers and nursery nurses who have specialist qualifications and skills that they use with under 8s	Working in schools, hospitals, nurseries and children's centres, planning the care and education of children under 8
Family support workers	No formal qualification needed but experience with families and children. May have NVQ in Child Care and Education	Working with families in the community to support children who are 'at risk' and may be on the Child Protection Register. Working with social workers attending case conferences and court hearings
Occupational therapists	Degree but there are opportunities to work as therapy assistants when a degree is not esstential	Helping people who have physical or mental health problems or disablties to help them cope with everyday life
Physiotherapists	Degree but there are opportunities to work as physiotherapy assistants when a degree is not essential	Helping people to regain physical ability after an operation or illness – like a stroke. Can work in hospital or in the community
Teachers (Early Years)	Degree in a national curriculum subject followed by a post-graduate teaching qualification, or a degree in education specialising in early years	Working in primary schools with responsibility for a class year and / or being responsible for a subject throughout the school, e.g. science

Table 2.4 (continued)

More details about jobs in the NHS are available on the website www.nhscareers. nhs.uk. It may be useful to look at the site as there are many careers in the NHS you may not have thought of before. Details about jobs in early years services can also be found on the Internet. Look at the www.direct.gov.uk/careers and you will find a range of jobs working with children.

Community psychiatric nurses

CPNs are employed by the Mental Health Trust and are concerned with supporting people with mental health problems in the community. However, they often work closely with their colleagues in hospital.

Nursing in hospital

Nursing posts in hospital can be in surgical or medical settings, in out-patients or in mental health care.

After you have completed your GCSE course, you may think about becoming a health care assistant (HCA) in a hospital.

ACTIVITY

Look at the following job description of a HCA in a busy London hospital. Look at it and decide what skills are required using Table 2.3.

Greenlands Hospital Trust Job Description:
Health Care Assistant
Functions

Patient care

1. Help with nursing care as instructed by nursing staff, including bathing, bed making, lifting patients and help with meals as necessary.
2. Caring for patients' personal clothing and other property in accordance with agreed policies relating to security and confidentiality.
3. Cleaning of beds and cleaning of lockers.

Ward responsibilities

1. Assisting the nursing staff to keep the ward tidy, including equipment and treatment rooms.
2. Assisting in checking, unpacking and storing of items delivered to the ward.
3. Answering the telephone and taking messages as required.
4. Being familiar with procedures related to health and safety, fire and other emergencies.

General

1. Observing complete confidentiality of information and records at all times, both on and off site.
2. Complying with all the Trust policies as they relate to staff, patients, relatives and visitors.
3. Undertaking errands as required.
4. Maintaining good working relations amongst staff.
5. Establishing and maintaining good relations with visitors and relatives, helping them to find their way around the hospital site.

In addition to medicine and nursing, there are a number of roles within the health care occupational area.

Allied Health Professionals (AHPs)

Examples of AHPs include the following:

- speech and language therapist
- occupational therapist
- radiographer
- radiotherapist.

These qualifications all require a three-year degree course at university, but there are also opportunities for people to work as assistants to these workers.

Figure 2.29 shows the range of jobs that are available in social care. At the moment, qualified social workers have a two-year diploma course or a degree in social work. The qualifications have been reviewed, and all qualifying programmes are likely to take three years in future.

Social workers can be employed in private organisations or by voluntary groups.

Social workers also work in hospitals, and this often involves liaising with other local council services for people returning home.

Social care assistant	No minimum requirements. Initial training given. NVQs available	Supporting users in their home and in the community Domiciliary care Residential care
Social worker	Degree or diploma	Can be based in community, attached to hospital or local council Supports a range of client groups – families, and children, mental health patients, disabled groups, older people

Table 2.5 Examples of qualifications needed for jobs in social care

Social care

Social care workers can include people with NVQs (National Vocational Qualifications) and other qualifications and also unqualified people. They usually work under the supervision of a qualified professional. Social care jobs are usually found in three main areas:

- domiciliary care (people being looked after in their own homes)
- residential care
- day care.

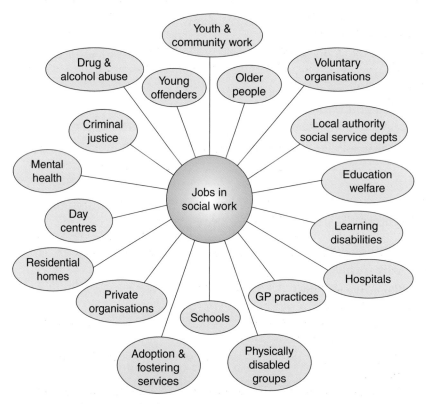

Figure 2.29 The range of jobs in social work

Here is the job description of a home carer, a person who looks after people in their own homes.

Department of Community Services Post: Home Carer

General Purpose of the Job

To provide seven-day personal care and domestic help to people living in their own homes. Service users will be older people, families with children, and people with a disability or mental illness, including those with carers such as relatives or friends. The post-holder will be a team member committed to providing a caring service which puts the user first.

Personal Care

1. Assist with day-to-day grooming, washing, bathing (parker bath only) and dressing, getting the user up and putting to bed.
2. Help with toileting, dealing with incontinence and catheter care, emptying and disinfecting commodes.
3. Assist with feeding, including preparation of meals and awareness of special dietary needs.
4. Administration of medication prescribed by the doctor, including applying creams and inserting eye drops.

Domestic duties – to be discussed and agreed with client

1. To undertake general housework, bed making and changing bed linen.
2. Washing personal clothing and household linen in user's home or local laundrette, or day centre.
3. Shop, pay bills, collect prescriptions and pensions.
4. Assist with financial affairs, keeping accurate records of all transactions.
5. Help with correspondence and letter writing.
6. Assist with pets.

General duties

1. Write detailed reports on user's progress and changes in their needs, behaviour or circumstances on a care plan in the user's home. To inform the team leader of any such changes.
2. Attend training sessions and meetings such as team meetings, case conferences and supervision sessions, as required.
3. Be responsible and handle emergencies with users in non-office hours, which may require the carer to make a decision to call medical or emergency aid.
4. Liaise with other professional involved with the user, e.g. GP, social worker, care manager, warden.
5. Accompany the user to pre-arranged appointments and occasional shopping trips, outings as required.
6. Carers may hold keys for their users and must be responsible for their safe keeping.
7. To establish a relationship with the user, give support to those under stress and provide companionship and a link with the community.
8. Work in accordance with department policies, practice and legislation relevant to their work, in particular, Health and Safety at Work and complaints.
9. Must carry out all duties in accordance with the Council's Equal Opportunities Policy.
10. Any other comparable duties required by the line manager.

ACTIVITY

Look at the Job Description and decide what qualities and skills are needed for the post using Table 2.3.

Job descriptions tend to focus on tasks that the worker has to do.

Caring for children

Workers in child care may have a range of qualifications. Figure 2.30 shows the main jobs looking after children.

Look at the job description of a nursery nurse working in a crèche attached to a hospital. What skills are required for this post?

Indirect carers

We have already seen examples of indirect carers on page 84.

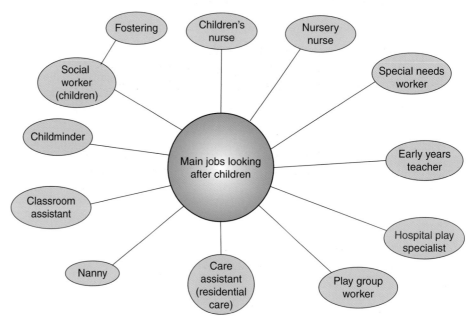

Figure 2.30 Jobs available working with children

Job Description: Nursery Nurse in the hospital crèche

Role
1. To be directly responsible for the general well-being of the children in the crèche and to satisfy their basic needs.
2. To carry out all professional duties as you may be required to do.
3. To maintain health and safety standards at all times.

Duties
1. To organise play facilities and to act in a caring role, i.e. changing, feeding and the care of clothing.
2. To ensure that any child who appears in any way unwell is removed from the crèche as soon as possible by the parent (or other responsible

(continued)

Job Description: Nursery Nurse in the hospital crèche – (continued)

   person nominated by the parent) and that the crèche manager is informed.

3. To discuss with the manager any child who is causing, or appears to have problems.

4. To see that the toys and play equipment are maintained in good order; that any faulty or potentially dangerous equipment is made immediately inaccessible to the children, and its condition reported to the most senior member of staff.

5. To be responsible for ordering toys and play equipment and at Christmas to assist with the selection and distribution of toys.

6. To be responsible for the overall tidiness and appearance of the crèche and to contribute to the general decorations.

7. To take the children for walks and other activities as appropriate, provided that permission is given by the parents.

Education and training

1. To assist in the instruction of all work experience students.

2. To maintain an-up-to date knowledge of developments in nursery nursing. This may include attending courses after discussion with the manager.

Safety

1. To be conversant with procedures carried out in case of accident.

2. To be conversant with procedures carried out in case of fire.

So far, we have looked at jobs that give direct care to patients in the community and in the hospital, but there are several workers in GP practices who give support to doctors and nurses.

Practice managers

These are key people in the practice, and are in charge of the receptionists, secretaries and other workers. They have overall responsibility for the smooth running of the surgery. They make sure that the computers are working, and make appointments for drug representatives to see the doctors. They ensure that all staff working in the practice are aware of health and safety issues. They interview new staff and provide an induction to the practice. They are responsible for the holiday rota system, and they deal with complaints from patients.

Practice managers have a wide range of backgrounds. They could have previous experience in social care or nursing, but they have to have good office skills. In order to become a practice manager, you have to take the Diploma in Practice Management.

Medical receptionist

A receptionist is the first person the patient comes into contact with when entering the surgery or when phoning with a query or to make an appointment. Many patients are very anxious when they call the receptionist. The receptionist must be careful to be aware of issues of confidentiality. If a patient telephones the surgery wanting to know the result of a test, there are usually clear guidelines about the correct procedure to be followed and the doctor will usually speak to the patient personally if there is an abnormal result. Receptionists may hear details of a private nature being discussed, and it is very important that these matters are not referred to elsewhere.

Figure 2.31 shows the organisation of a health centre.

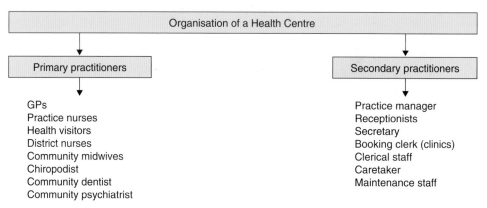

Figure 2.31 Organisation chart of a health centre

Indirect carers also work in schools and hospitals

School reception staff

All schools have reception staff who work in the school office. They are responsible for keeping records of children and doing clerical work. They will also need to have IT skills as most records are now kept on a computer. They may help with open evenings and other events that are held by the school. They need to be calm and able to cope with parents who may be concerned about the progress their child is making at school. They may deal with minor accidents in the playground. They also need to keep information about children confidential.

Catering staff

Catering staff are responsible for the provision of meals to children. They may cook food on the premises or the food may be delivered from a central kitchen. Great importance is given to preparing, serving and storing food safely. Most catering staff have to have a Food Hygiene certificate, and they may also be encouraged to take part in first aid training. Catering staff may be employed by the school or they may belong to an agency that provides the service to the school.

Indirect services that are usually outsourced to private companies

The indirect services that are provided in hospitals have already been outlined earlier in this chapter. Agencies that provide these services may provide training in cleaning and catering.

Security staff

Security staff are used in hospitals and these are usually provided by outside agencies. Security staff patrol the hospital premises and grounds and make sure that no unauthorised people are in the area. They may also have to deal with incidents such as drunk and abusive patients in A and E. They may have previous experience in the police, fire service or armed forces. They need to be able to cope with unexpected events, such as fire alarms or other emergencies.

Portering

This is another important service that may be provided by agencies. Porters need to be physically fit and able to communicate effectively with patients and staff. They also need a good sense of direction to find their way round a large hospital! They are responsible for taking patients to theatre on trolleys; or taking patients in wheelchairs to different departments in the hospital for x-rays and other investigations, as well as moving equipment. They may also have to transport patients who have died to the mortuary.

Waste management

Waste management is an essential part of work in hospitals, surgeries and care homes. There are two types of waste.

Clinical waste from health care that can include the following:

- material contaminated with human tissue or body fluids
- sharp objects such as discarded syringe needles or broken glass
- medicines
- chemical waste.

In many care settings the amount of waste may be small, but in hospitals it will be a large quantity.

Hazardous waste

Waste that may be harmful to human health or to the environment.

Care staff have a responsibility to dispose of waste carefully. Clinical waste is put in yellow bags for disposal and 'sharps' needles or syringes are placed in an approved container.

There are laws about the safe disposal of waste. Records must be kept to show that waste is properly disposed of. In hospitals, care homes and surgeries an approved clinical waste collector is used to remove waste.

Care values which underpin service provider interaction

In this section we will look at the care values that underpin service provider interaction

Care values which underpin care practice with service users

Health and social care and early years practitioners need to understand the importance of the care values that underpin the service they give to service users.

Health and care practitioners use guidelines and codes of practice to empower clients by:

- promoting anti-discriminatory practice
- promoting and supporting individual rights to dignity, independence, health and safety
- promoting effective communication and relationships
- maintaining confidentiality of information
- acknowledging individual personal beliefs and identity
- maintaining confidentiality
- promoting individual rights and beliefs.

Care values are the basic tool used to empower and encourage trusting relationships between client and carer. These values underpin the work of all professional carers and these values are derived from Human Rights. Health and social care practitioners need to show their clients that they value him or her as an individual and the care that is given promotes equality and cultural diversity.

Promoting anti-discriminatory practice

People may discriminate without realising it, but as care workers we must be careful not to use stereotypes when supporting patients and clients. At the same time, we need to be aware that everyone is an individual and we are not effective care workers if we treat everyone the same.

Discriminatory behaviour can include:

- racist and sexist jokes
- isolating clients with a mental health problem
- avoiding looking after someone who is from a different ethnic background from your own
- ignoring the needs of someone with HIV
- excluding certain residents from activities.

Discriminatory behaviour can also be indicated through:

- tone of voice (loud and aggressive)
- body language (distant and threatening)
- eye gaze (avoiding eye contact, or glaring).

Most health and social care organisations have an equal opportunities policy.

If you go on work experience try to look at the equal opportunities policy at the placement.

Promoting and supporting individual rights to dignity, independence, health and safety

In health and social care the rights of clients and patients are often stated in policies and charters. Here is an example of a charter of rights found in an older people's residential home.

CHARTER of RIGHTS

As a resident of this Home you should enjoy the following rights:

Your Room
- To have privacy by locking your room door and any cupboards inside your room.
- To have access to your own room when you wish.
- To entertain visitors in your room and to invite people to visit you whenever you wish. If you share a room, it is customary to ask the other occupant.

The Home
- To choose how you spend your day and who you spend your day with. You may wish simply to be alone.
- To eat when you wish during specified meal times.
- To select your meals from a choice on the menu.

(continued)

CHARTER of RIGHTS

**As a resident of this Home you should enjoy
the following rights: – (continued)**

- To assist in preparing the Home's menu.
- To use the Home's facilities for preparing snacks and beverages.
- To choose your bathing and washing times and who, if anyone, gives you support.
- To rise and go to bed when you please.
- To take part in any social and recreational activities that are organised.
- To contribute to the running of the Home by attending residents' committee meetings.
- To have influence over the spending of the Home's Amenity Fund through majority voting with other residents.
- To use the pay phone at any time for your private use.

Think about where you live at the moment. Can you do the activities the residents in this home can?

Most residential homes have a similar charter.

If you have work experience you can find out about the rights of clients by looking at:

- codes of practice
- staff policies
- charters and other policies for service users
- standards of care.

Although it is important to respect the values of clients and patients, you also need to be aware of the rights of other clients and service users, and of safety issues.

In order to promote anti-discriminatory practice, health and care organisations should:

- develop policies
- implement the policies
- give staff training in promoting better care to all clients
- have a complaints procedure so that patients and clients can have their say.

All care workers find they like some of their patients more than others. This is natural. What you need to ask yourself is why you do not like a client? Is it because you feel awkward dealing with them because you do not understand their religion or culture? Finding out about their views may be beneficial for everyone.

Promoting individual rights and beliefs

These are some examples of legislation that promotes individuals rights and beliefs.

- **The Race Relations Act (1976)**
  This Act bans all forms of racial discrimination in work, housing and the provision of services. The Act has been revised to include indirect discrimination (Race Relations Amendment Act 2000).

- The Sex Discrimination Act (1975)

  This Act makes it unlawful to discriminate on the grounds of sex. Sex discrimination is unlawful in employment, education, advertising or when providing housing, goods or services or facilities. It is unlawful to discriminate because someone is married. It is unlawful to discriminate in advertising for jobs.

- Disability Discrimination Act (1995)

  This Act gives rights to disabled people in employment, access to education and transport, housing and obtaining goods and services. In the Disability Discrimination Amendment Act (2005) public bodies (like councils) have a positive duty to promote equality for disabled people.

Direct Discrimination is an act which deliberately excludes a certain group on the basis of gender, race, age, or sexuality.

If a landlord puts up a notice in the window for a lodger and says 'No Irish or Blacks' you can see that this is a clear example of direct discrimination and it would be illegal to do this nowadays.

Indirect discrimination is more complex.

What do you think of this advertisement?

> 'Driver wanted for old people's home. Must be able to lift heavy items, have English at GCSE standard and be 6 feet tall.'

Although the advert doesn't clearly state it wants white males, the personal factors required make this likely. Not many women are 6 feet tall, and workers who have English as a second language are less likely to have GCSE at the standard stated. If the advertiser was challenged over this advert, he/she would have to prove that the height and English qualification were needed for the job.

Individuals rights and beliefs

What do we mean by the term rights? Think for a moment what you understand to be your rights.

- Rights can be covered by laws, e.g. the right to drive a car at 17, the right to vote, or get married.
- Rights can also been seen as natural or as universal rights, e.g. the right to work, the right to have children, the right to make choices about what you do in your daily life.

Human Rights Act (1998)

This Act covers a range of human rights that affects health and care practice. The following Articles are the most relevant:

Article 2 – Everyone's life shall be protected by law.

Article 3 – No one should be subjected to torture or to inhuman or degrading treatment or punishment.

Article 5 – Everyone has the right to liberty and security of their person.

Article 6 – Everyone is entitled to a fair and public hearing in any civil or criminal matter.

Article 8 – Everyone has the right to respect for their private and family life, their home and correspondence.

Article 9 – Everyone has the right to freedom of thought, conscience and religion.

Article 10 – Everyone has the right to freedom of expression.

Article 12 – Men and women of marriageable age have the right to marry and have a family.

Article 14 – The enjoyment of rights and freedoms should be secured without discrimination on any grounds such as sex, race, colour, language, religion, political or other opinion, national or social origin, association with a national minority, property, birth or other status.

ACTIVITY

Look at the following care issues and identify which Article is most relevant (in some instances there could be more than one possibility).

1. Peter, who has Downs Syndrome, lives in sheltered accommodation. If he wants to withdraw money from his bank account he has to have the signature of his key worker.

2. Maria, who has a mild learning disability, wants to start living with her boyfriend.

3. Craig has a disagreement over the level of care he is receiving. His GP decides he wants to remove him from his list of patients.

4. Surita, who is a wheelchair user, wants to have a baby, but when she talks about this to her care worker, she is discouraged.

5. Richard has a long-standing mental health problem. He has a crisis and he is admitted to hospital as a compulsory patient (this is called sectioning). It is decided he needs to have an Electro-Convulsive Therapy (ECT) and also heavy sedation.

6. A recent report in a local paper highlights the widespread use of tranquilizers in nursing homes to keep patients quiet and easy to deal with.

As you can see, the Human Rights Act links into the care value base and may have an important effect on the way health and care issues are resolved.

Examples of discriminatory practice in health and social care could include the following:

- a nursery that refuses to take a child with HIV
- a nursery that refuses to take a child who has a facial disfigurement, saying it will frighten the other children
- a teenager with Downs Syndrome who cannot find a dentist willing to take him on his list
- a refugee who cannot find a GP to take him on as a patient.

People are treated unfairly because of prejudice and the use of stereotypes that are often reinforced by the media.

For example, the stereotype of older people is that they are all deaf and act like children.

As we have already seen a stereotype is:

'a fixed idea of a particular person or group. If you stereotype people you expect them all to behave in a particular way'.

This can be reinforced through television and the media, so that, unless you have personal experience of older people, when you care for an older person you may shout at them (they are deaf) and suggest activities for them to do such as playing musical chairs (they act like children).

There are many examples of codes of practice. Codes of conduct for social workers cover the key principles of care.

Social workers must, to the best of their ability:

- protect the rights and promote the interests of service users and carers
- strive to establish and maintain the trust and confidence of services users and carers
- promote the independence of service users while protecting them as far as possible from danger or harm
- respect the rights of services users while seeking to ensure that their behaviour does not harm themselves or other people
- be accountable for the quality of their work and take responsibility for maintaining and improving their knowledge and skills

(taken from the General Social Care Council website www.gscc.org.uk).

The full document is available on this website.

Policies for staff

Nowadays most organisations have a range of policies. These can include:

- health and safety
- equal opportunities
- confidentiality
- complaints policies and procedures.

These policies give guidelines to staff, but also indicate how patients' and clients' rights should be protected.

If you go on work experience try to find some examples of policies.

Standards in health care

All NHS (including PCTs) Trusts have a PALS department which deals with comments and complaints and all complaints have to be recorded and publicised in the Annual Report.

The Health Care Commission (the Commission for Healthcare Audit and Inspection) is the organisation that inspects hospitals (both NHS and private) to make sure that patients' services are at a good standard. They make sure that patient dignity is respected. The inspectors talk to patients and staff and produce a report that is available on their website www.healthcarecommission. org.uk.

When you register with your GP you have a right:

- to be offered a health check when you join a practice for the first time
- to ask for a health check-up if you are between 16 and 74 and have not seen the GP for the last three years
- be offered an annual health check in the GPs surgery, or at your own home if you prefer, if you are 75 or over.

KEY TERM

PALS – this stands for Patient Advice and Liaison Service. This service advises patients when they are concerned about anything to do with their health care in the Trust.

Standards in social care

Local authorities have contracts with voluntary and other independent organisations, and as part of the service agreement the organisation has to provide care that reaches a certain standard. Social services also produce standards of service statements that tell clients what service they can expect.

The Commission for Social Care Inspection – Residential Homes have to be registered with CSCI and inspectors make announced and unannounced visits. If a relative or resident is unhappy with the care at a home they can contact CSCI and report the matter. The CSCI has the powers to close homes that are unsatisfactory.

The client has rights to dignity. When CSCI inspectors visit a residential home, they talk to residents and relatives to find out if the clients are treated with respect. They would expect the following practice:

- staff will knock on the door before entering (and wait for an answer)
- staff will address clients by the name they choose
- the privacy of the client will be respected.

Promoting effective communication and relationships

Clare is a practice nurse at a doctors' surgery. It is Tuesday morning and she sees that the following patients have booked in to see her.

Mrs Brown (80) who needs to have her ears syringed; she lives on her own and is a frequent visitor to the surgery.

Tom Bell (35) – he has had a knee operation and he needs his dressing changed.

Charlotte Evans (25) who is booked to have an assessment of her asthma.

Ted Phillips (65) who is in a wheelchair after a stroke and needs a blood test.

Narinda Patel (55) who is being monitored for her blood pressure.

Tom Dodwell (7) who has fallen off his bike in the woods and needs a tetanus injection. He has come with his mother.

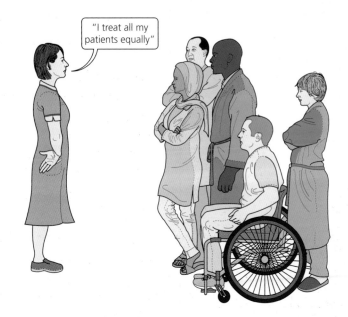

"I treat all my patients equally"

Figure 2.32 What are the problems with the nurse's attitude?

ACTIVITY

It may be interesting to look at the website and see if you can find the latest report on your local hospital.

ACTIVITY

In your groups discuss each patient in turn.

How should Clare approach them?

Would she approach each patient in the same way?

What needs may they have that Clare should take into account when she sees them?

DISCUSSION

You may have thought of such things as:

● approaching each person; do you use the same language to a person who is 7 or is 80?
● what cultural aspects may you need to be aware of; for example, if Narinda is vegetarian and she is being advised on a diet to help her blood pressure you need to be aware of this
● how do you think someone in a wheelchair likes to be spoken to?
● if someone has had a stroke it may affect their speech; how would you approach Ted?

Communication skills do not just include listening and talking, they also include non-verbal communication.

ACTIVITY

1. Working with a partner, move your chairs so you cannot see each other. Without turning round, take it in turns to talk to each other, one acting as speaker, the other acting as listener. The one acting as listener is not allowed to say anything, and that includes grunting and laughing. When you have finished, discuss how you felt as a listener and as a talker.
2. Sitting face to face, take it in turns to act as a listener and talker. This time the listener avoids looking at the speaker during their conversation. How does this feel?

Non-verbal communication

Non-verbal communication is communication without words. The following are examples of non-verbal communication:

● physical contact – touching, holding hands, hugging, etc.
● proximity – how close you sit or stand when you are talking to people
● posture – how you stand or sit, crossed arms, crossed legs, leaning forward
● gestures – what you do with your hands and arms, also nodding or shaking your head
● facial expression – smiling, laughing, frowning
● eye contact and movement – staring, blinking, winking, looking at someone
● tone of voice – loud, soft, aggressive
● pace of voice – speaking fast, slowly, hesitating.

The reasons why you found the first exercise uncomfortable in the activity is that we look at the person we are talking to in order to gain a response, and we can respond using non-verbal communication as well to reinforce the communication process.

The second exercise also demonstrates the importance of eye contact when communicating with someone.

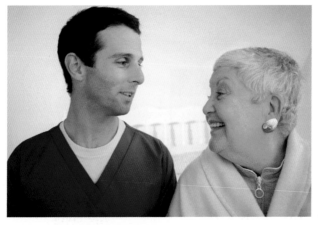
Figure 2.33 Philip and Mrs Tate

ACTIVITY

Look at Figure 2.33. This shows a photograph of Philip, a volunteer worker, talking to a client at a day centre. Make a list of non-verbal communication you can see.

Philip is looking at Mrs Tate; he is smiling and he is sitting in his chair at the same level at Mrs Tate. Another interesting thing we can see here is that Philip is reflecting Mrs Tate's facial expressions.

This is called mirroring, and is often done unconsciously when people are trying to establish an equal relationship.

Next time you are in a café, or in the college dining room, make a note of the non-verbal communication you can see occurring between two people. Not only may you see facial expressions mirrored, but you may see other gestures reflected by the couples, such as touching their own hair, hand movements, etc. We need to be aware of non-verbal communication, and also how some forms of verbal communication may be appropriate in some situations and not in others.

As you can see, it isn't just the words you say that are important, but tone of voice, posture, facial expression, and gestures. On the phone, the tone of voice is very important, and you also have to speak more clearly and slowly as the person you are speaking to cannot see you for additional non-verbal information.

If you become impatient or aggressive with an aggressive patient or client, the situation can get worse, so it is important to keep calm before you say anything.

Useful strategies:

- If something isn't clear, ask for additional information. Sometimes this slows down the communication and can reduce tension.
- Take a deep breath and speak slowly and clearly.
- Maintain eye contact if face to face, and try to sit down rather than stand up, as people are more relaxed if they are sitting down. If the patient is in bed or in a chair, make sure you are at the same level, rather than standing over them.
- Respect issues of confidentiality.
- Don't try to score points or put people down.

Benefits of effective communication

- The care worker can obtain and provide useful information that is relevant to clients'/patients' well-being.
- It enables the care worker to support and understand the client/patient.
- It assists teamwork.
- It can help patients make their needs known.

If communication is not effective:

- patients can feel angry and resentful
- patients feel they are not being listened to and understood
- patients don't understand why certain procedures are happening
- patients may not follow treatment and exercise that may help them recover.

Physical contact

Health and social care workers often touch patients and clients in order to show support and understanding. Look at Figure 2.34. The photograph shows Ashna,

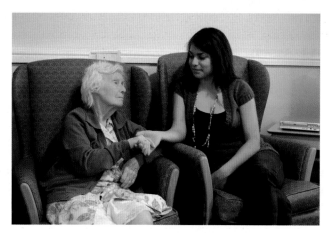

Figure 2.34 Ashna and Mrs Gibson

a care worker at a day centre, with a client. Note the non-verbal communication that is shown by the people in the photograph. You can see that Ashna is holding Mrs Gibson's hand. Why do you think she is doing this? Would you think it was appropriate if Ashna was a male carer? As care workers we need to be aware of the appropriate use of touch, especially on different parts of the body. The hands and arms are usually seen as acceptable areas to touch, but to touch other parts of the body, such as thigh, neck or knee, would be seen as off-limits unless you are massaging or washing someone. Again, there are cultural differences. Asian women would not wish to be touched by a man. Because of problems of accusations of abuse, all care workers need to be aware of the appropriate use of touch.

Written communication

> ### ACTIVITY
>
> Write down all the examples of written communication you would use in health and social care.

In health and social care work, written communication is very important.

Your list could include:

- patient records
- care plans
- referral letters
- accident report forms
- prescriptions
- consent forms.

Patients' records are legal documents and could be used in a court of law. It is important they are:

- clear
- easy to read
- concise
- based on fact and not on opinion.

Nowadays many records are being kept in electronic form on the computer. This is important for information such as the discharge summary when a patient leaves hospital. The patient or carer will be given a copy, which is more helpful than trying to remember what the doctor or nurse said to them.

ACTIVITY

Consider these two examples of a patient record of Mrs Brown who is on the medical ward.

EXAMPLE A

Mrs Brown had a good night.

EXAMPLE B

Mrs Brown slept for six hours without medication. She woke up at 6 am and said she was free from pain, and did not require a pain killer.

DISCUSSION

In Example A, 'a good night,' could mean anything. It is vague and does not give any information.

In Example B, we know that Mrs Brown slept for six hours; she was not in pain, and did not need a painkiller. The use of Mrs Brown's own words is also seen as a reliable record.

Other forms of communication

Other forms of communication used in health and social care can include:

- posters (often to do with health promotion)
- leaflets
- diagrams.

When communicating with children, leaflets may be too complicated, and diagrams may be more appropriate.

Figure 2.35 is an example of a record kept by a child who is attending an enuresis clinic (for bedwetting). The child colours in the appropriate box. It is clear and gives an encouraging message to the child. It is also easy for the nurse to check the progress that is being made.

The differing communication needs of client groups in health and social care

Difficulty in speaking

There are several groups of people who have difficulty speaking. This could be due to problems from birth, such as cerebral palsy, or difficulties in later life due to accidents or strokes. According to the Stroke Association, every five minutes someone in England and Wales has a stroke. Ten thousand people each year have speech problems as a result of a stroke. The Stroke Association runs programmes for people who have aphasia (difficulty speaking). Speech and language therapists

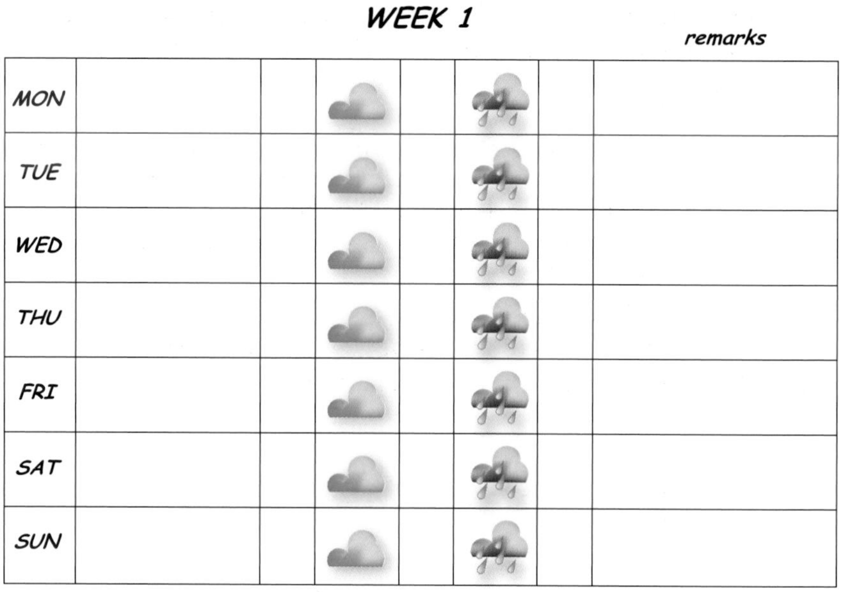

WEEK 1

remarks

MON			☁		🌧	
TUE			☁		🌧	
WED			☁		🌧	
THU			☁		🌧	
FRI			☁		🌧	
SAT			☁		🌧	
SUN			☁		🌧	

Figure 2.35 An example of a record kept by a child

work with aphasic patients. The Stroke Association also produces visual aids (that patients can use, so that they can communicate by pointing at the relevant picture).

Here are some dos and don'ts for when you are communicating with someone who has a speech difficulty.

1. Do not finish the person's sentence for them.
2. Give them plenty of time.
3. If you are not clear what they have said, ask them to repeat it.
4. Use picture cards, computers or other communication means.
5. Do not forget that the person can still hear, even if they cannot speak clearly.

Maintaining confidentiality of information

Confidentiality is about keeping information private when it should be kept private. Think about the last time you went to see your doctor or practice nurse. What information would you be happy to give? What information would you feel uncomfortable about giving? How would you feel if your personal details were freely available to everyone?

A health and social care worker will know a great deal about the person they are looking after. It is essential that the information is kept confidential and not passed on without the client's permission.

Some information may have to be passed on from one care worker to another, or from a nurse to a doctor, but this must be done with the patient's permission.

The death of a patient does not give you the right to break confidentiality.

The Code: Standards of conduct, performance and ethics for nurses and midwives states the following:

Respect for confidentiality

- you must respect people's right to confidentiality
- you must ensure people are informed how and why information is shared by those who will be providing their care

- you must disclose information if you believe someone may be at risk of harm, in line with the law of the country in which you are practising.

(Nursing and Midwifery Council www.nmc-uk.org)

Confidentiality can only be broken in exceptional circumstances. Every health and caring organisation will have a policy on confidentiality and the disclosure of information. Patients and clients have a right to know that their personal details are kept private and confidential. If you, as the care worker, need to disclose information this should be done:

- with the consent of the client or patient
- without the consent of the client or patient if required by law
- without the consent of the client or patient if the disclosure is seen to be in the public interest.

ACTIVITY

Example 1

You are on night duty on the children's ward. One of the children tells you her step-father is abusing her. What do you do?

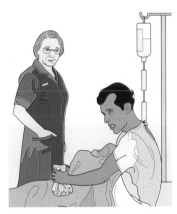

Figure 2.36 Nurses have to make difficult decisions

Example 2

You are working on a male medical ward. A young man is brought in as an emergency. He has a bag with him that he asks you to keep in a safe place. He tells you that he has just arrived from India, and he is taking Schedule A drugs to his brother. He asks you to keep his secret.

DISCUSSION

In both these examples the duty of the nurse is quite clear, as in both cases it is a matter of public interest, but a lot of cases are quite difficult, and you would need to discuss them with your manager. In the two examples given, you would first report the matter to your line manager.

Written records

Medical records are also covered by the same principles of confidentiality. There are usually procedures for keeping records safe in locked filing cabinets.

The 1987 Access to Personal Files Act allows patients to see their personal medical or social service files from this date. Notice to view your records is required. Doctors charge a fee for this service, and any record that may be damaging to the patient (in the opinion of the doctor) can be withheld. People with mental health problems could come into this category.

Computer-based records

Many hospitals and surgeries now keep records on computer. The Data Protection Act (1984) covers all information that is held about people on computers. Every organisation that holds computer-based records must be registered, and there are guidelines for good practice that have to be followed.

1. The information must have been obtained legally and without deceit.
2. The information should only be used for the purpose for which it was collected.
3. The information should not be disclosed to anyone who has no right to see it.
4. There should be a proper security system, with a password require

Confidentiality is a key aspect in all health and social care work.

Acknowledging individual personal beliefs and identity

In a multi-cultural society it is very important that health, social care and early years workers have a good understanding of the cultures of different client groups. The different cultural groups may differ from other groups in the following ways:

- family organisation
- the roles of men and women
- the attitudes to professional health and social care workers
- dress/clothing
- language
- personal care
- diet
- preparing for pregnancy and childbirth
- preparing for death – and afterwards
- religious practice.

Culture is not just about language; it is about all those other aspects of daily life that are part of the way of life for some groups in UK society

Many people who live in large cities in the UK have English as a second language, and when these people have to access health and social care services interpreters are needed.

In order for the interpreter to be effective he or she must:

- have knowledge of the subject matter – it could be quite complicated if treatment or benefits are being discussed
- build up trust with the client so that they can reach a good level of understanding about their concerns
- have a good understanding of the cultural issues of the client
- be appropriate to the needs of the client – this would include the gender and age of the interpreter and the client. Many Asian women would not feel comfortable with a male interpreter.

If you are looking after someone who has limited English you could use:

- signs /drawings to tell the patient about their care
- hand movements and signals – a bit like charades – but this could be embarrassing for both of you!

KEY TERMS

Translators – a translator works with the written word so they are useful when you need to present information in leaflets and posters that can be understood by different groups and also in all other written communications. An organisation called Multikulti translates leaflets and information in a wide range of languages. Their website is www.multikulti.org.uk. You may find it interesting to look at.

Interpreters – are people who communicate the meaning of what is said from one language to another.

- non-verbal communication to reassure the patient
- short sentences and simple words.

CASE STUDY 3

In West London there was a concern about the low number of Bangladeshi women attending the antenatal clinic at the hospital. Anne, the community midwife, visited the patients at their homes, but often the door was not answered, although she was sure someone was at home. At the clinic, she tried to explain to women that she needed a urine sample from them – this produced a lot of embarrassment. An Asian Link Worker scheme was set up and the Link Worker visited patients in their homes with Anne and attended the clinic. The worker explained to the women what was needed and why, and she also explained to Anne how the Bangladeshi women felt about Anne. The women tended to look away from Anne when she was talking to them and she thought they were being moody, but the worker explained to Anne that in their culture looking away from someone, rather than looking them straight in the eye was a sign of respect.

If we are part of a multi-cultural society it is important that all our organisations provide information in other languages, as well as providing English lessons for those who are now part of the UK. Nurseries, schools, hospitals and care organisations must all provide support for people who have English as a second language.

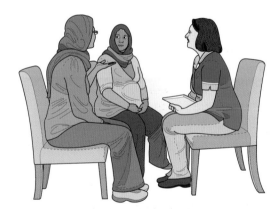

Figure 2.37 Effective communication is essential in a multi-cultural society

How these care values are reflected in the behaviour, attitudes and work of care practitioners

The Every Child Matters Agenda

So far in this section we have looked at the care values that underpin all services.

However, practitioners who work with children and young people have particular responsibilities under the Every Child Matters recommendations. We have already seen that social services now have a separate children's department following the Children Act.

KEY TERM

Empowerment – all care practitioners should support their clients/patients so that they can make decisions about all aspects of their care and they are involved in planning their care.

OFSTED (the Office for Standards in Education) is the organisation that is responsible for inspecting all children's services such as nurseries, childminders and children's social services.

Although these guidelines were for people working with children and young people we can find them helpful when looking at other kinds of care:

- care of older people, either in their own home or in residential care
- care of people with learning difficulties
- care of people with mental health needs
- care of people with disabilities.

In all these client groups we need to balance the importance of encouraging independence through empowering people we work with, with the risks that we need to think about.

In this chapter we have seen how care workers can use communication methods so that clients and patients can be supported. It's important that the behaviour, attitudes and work of care practitioners reflects the care values. This aspect of caring is discussed again in Chapter 4.

ACTIVITY

Look at the following list of requirements of the Every Child Matters and discuss how these standards also apply to all patients and client groups we have discussed so far.

- make the welfare of the child paramount – this means that the child's interests must come first, and central to all planned care
- keep children safe and maintain a healthy environment – this means that the child is protected from abuse or other dangers, both from others and from the environment, such as the nursery
- work in partnership with families and parents – this means the main care giver is involved in deciding on and giving care
- make sure that children are offered a range of experiences and activities that supports all their development – this means children are able to play and do other activities that support their intellectual, social and physical development
- value diversity; children may be the same age in a group but they are all different – in gender, culture, language, religion so they must be treated accordingly
- promote equal opportunity – it is important that child care workers give all the children in their care equal access to activities, education and experiences
- maintain confidentiality – as we have already seen, it is important to keep information about children in your care confidential
- ensure anti-discriminatory practice – child care workers must not treat one child more favourably than the others in their care because of prejudice or stereotyping
- work with others – since the Children Act, partnerships have been developed between all those involved in child care including the police as well as health and social care workers and teachers in schools
- are a reflective practitioner – this is about thinking about what we do as carers and how we can improve our practice; this could be through going on additional training courses or discussing our clients with other members of the team

GLOSSARY

Absolute poverty – a lack of resources sufficient to maintain a healthy existence

Abuse – treating people badly, either physically or emotionally

Chronic condition – a disease of long duration involving very slow changes; it often starts very gradually

Cohabitation – a couple living together who are not married or in a civil partnership

Culture – shared values based on beliefs, practice, dress, language , diet and religion

Discrimination – the unfair treatment of a person, or group, because of a negative view of some, or all, of their characteristics (could be based on ethnicity, gender or age).

Disease – a specific condition of ill health, identified as an actual change on the surface or inside some part of the body.

Emotional health – concerned with being able to express feelings such as fear, joy, grief, frustration and anger. It also includes the ability to cope with anxiety, stress, and depression

Ethnicity – a shared identity which comes from a common culture, religion or tradition

Gender – the psychological and social development of male and female roles in a society

Homophobia – fear and hatred of homosexuals

Ideal self – the type of person you would most like to be

Identity – self image; how you see yourself and what you know about yourself

Illness – the subjective state of feeling unwell (i.e. how people feel). (Compare with Disease and Sickness)

Intellectual health – concerned with the ability to think clearly and rationally; it is closely linked to emotional and social health

Menopause – when women stop menstruating

Nuclear family – family consisting of one woman and one man with dependent children

Physical health – concerned with the physical functioning of the body. It is the easiest aspect of health to measure.

Poverty – lack of resources helping you to be healthy

Primary relationship – close relationship based on kinship. marriage, adoption, friendship or blood ties

Redundancy – when work or a job no longer exists for the worker who is then made unemployed

Relative poverty – a lack of resources (income) sufficient to achieve a standard of living considered acceptable in a society

Role model – an example of behaviour or achieved status in society that is seen as good

Secondary relationship – more distant or formal relationship that may be short term

Self-concept – how you see yourself as a separate individual

Self-image (identity) – how you see yourself and what you know about yourself

GLOSSARY – (continued)

Self-esteem – the value you place on yourself

Self-fulfilling prophecy – a belief that things turn out as you predict because people behave in such a way as to bring about the prediction- usually to do with behaviour

Sibling – brother or sister

Sickness – reported illness; involves being treated by a professional and becoming a medical statistic.

Social health – this is concerned with the ability to relate to others and to form relationships

Social role – the way you behave in certain situations, such as student, nurse, etc

Socialisation – the way you learn as a child how to fit into society using the social skills and values of that society

Status – your social position related to others so may be high or low; is linked to factors such as wealth, income, social class, job, age and appearance

Stereotype – a simplified general image about a particular group of people, e.g. 'they all do that'

Working relationship – relationship based in working environment that is more distant or formal

Promoting Health and Well-Being

CHAPTER CONTENT

Health, social care and early years practitioners aim to promote the health and well-being of service users.

This chapter will help you develop knowledge and understanding of:
- definitions of health and well-being
- factors which affect health and well-being
- the effects of factors affecting health and well-being
- methods used to measure individual physical health
- ways of promoting and supporting health improvement

Understanding health and well-being

Different methods used by practitioners and individuals to define health and well being

There are several different ways of thinking about health and well-being.

'At least I've still got my health.' When someone says this, what do they mean by health? It is likely that you understand their meaning, but it is difficult for you to define the word 'health'. Different people will have different ideas about health. There is a range of definitions of health and well-being used by ordinary people, professionals and different organisations.

ACTIVITY

1. Before you read any further, think how you would define 'being healthy'. Ask a few of your friends what definition they would give.
2. Now read about the three types of definitions of health – negative, positive or holistic – and decide into which categories your definition falls.

There are three different definitions of health commonly given.

i) Holistic definition of health and well-being

'Health and well-being are the result of a combination of physical, social, intellectual and emotional factors.'

KEY TERM

Holistic – looking at the whole system rather than just concentrating on individual components.

A widely used definition of health came from the World Health Organisation (WHO) in 1948. This defines health as:

> 'a state of complete physical, mental and social well-being and not merely the absence of disease or infirmity'

This has been widely quoted because it goes much further than just seeing health as freedom from disease. Instead, health is viewed as all-round well-being (see Figure 3.1).

However, this definition has been criticised for two main reasons.

1. It is seen as too idealistic. How often do you really feel yourself to be in a state of 'complete well-being'?
2. It does not consider the ability to adapt to the changes that we all face throughout life. In the light of these criticisms, a more recent WHO definition of health is:

> 'The extent to which an individual or group is able, on the one hand, to realise aspirations and satisfy needs and, on the other hand, to change or cope with the environment. Health is a positive concept emphasising social and personal resources as well as physical capabilities.' (1984)

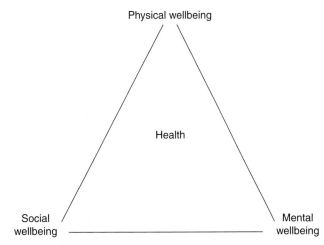

Figure 3.1 WHO definition of health (1948)

This definition shows that:

- health is an important part of our everyday lives
- health is a positive concept
- health is a much wider concept than freedom from disease
- health takes into account the whole person
- health is related to our ability to cope and adapt to change
- health might be understood in different ways by different individuals and groups.

Physical, intellectual, emotional and social health

The WHO definitions are holistic definitions as they encourage the view of health as concerned with the whole person and not just their physical state. When thinking about a person's health you should think about *p*hysical, *i*ntellectual, *e*motional and *s*ocial aspects (see Figure 3.2). You will be able to remember these if you think of the word 'PIES'.

Remember that these different aspects of health are not separate but overlap and influence one another. For example, the pain and discomfort of an illness may make you unhappy. In this case, your physical health is influencing your emotional health.

ii) Positive definitions of health and well-being

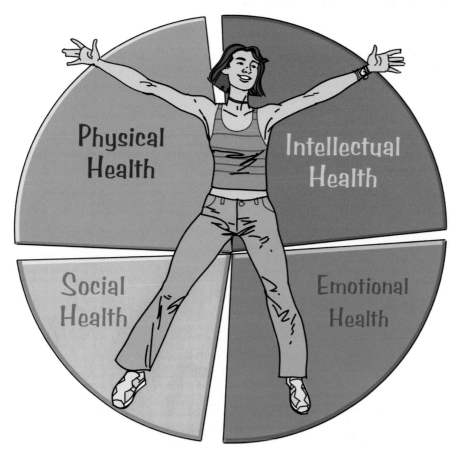

Figure 3.2 Holistic definition of health

'The achievement and maintenance of physical fitness and mental stability'

Some people think more positively of health as fitness and well-being. They may associate health with moods and feelings, and a sense of balance.

iii) Negative definitions of health and well-being

'The absence of physical illness, disease and mental distress'.

Many people only think about health when they are thinking about illness or health problems. This means they may give a negative definition of health, such as 'not being ill' or 'being free of pain'.

The medical definition of health is often thought to be 'absence of disease'. This is a negative definition. It does not describe health as a positive state. It views health as being when you are not classified as sick or in need of medical help. It ignores the fact that health is about feeling well, energetic and at ease. It may also mean that people with disabilities or chronic conditions (see glossary) may be labelled as 'sick' or 'diseased' when they are otherwise healthy.

KEY TERMS

Physical health – concerned with the physical functioning of the body. Physical health is the easiest aspect of health to measure.

Intellectual health – concerned with the ability to think clearly and rationally. It is closely linked to emotional and social health (see below).

Emotional health – concerned with the ability to recognise emotions such as fear, joy, grief, frustration and anger, and to express such emotions appropriately. Emotional health also includes the ability to cope with anxiety, stress and depression.

Social health – concerned with the ability to relate to others and to form relationships with other people.

ACTIVITY

1. Look at the glossary at the end of this chapter to check the meaning of illness, disease, and sickness.
2. Think about occasions on which you have been unwell and decide whether these episodes would have been classed as illness, disease, or sickness.

Different ideas about health and well-being

People have different standards of what being healthy means to them, depending on their life stage and cultural setting (Figure 3.3).

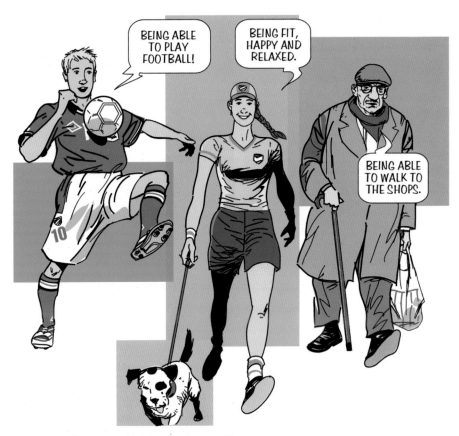

Figure 3.3 Different standards of being healthy

This may depend on:

- **Life stage (age)** – ideas about health and well-being change over time. For example, a young person might only consider they are healthy if they can take part in active sports, but an elderly person may consider themselves healthy if they can walk a short distance. From middle age onwards, people are more likely to think of mental well-being as well as physical well-being.
- **Culture** – people from certain cultures may have ideas about health which are different from a typical Western approach. For example, Hindus believe that illness is caused by the elements being out of harmony with the body. Treatment may include diet, massages and herbal cures to restore balance.

Muslims believe the body has four humours which are out of balance when a person is ill. They may be treated with yoga, diet or massage.

These examples show that ordinary people have a very subjective, not objective, view of health.

Factors affecting health and well-being

What factors affect an individual's health and well-being?

A person's health and well-being is affected by a number of different factors throughout their lives, in either a positive or negative way. The factors may be:

- physical
- social, cultural and emotional
- economic
- environmental
- psychological.

There is a summary of these factors in Figure 1.13 in Chapter 1 on page 21.

Physical factors

Genetic inheritance

(See also '*Genetic inheritance*' on page 22 in Chapter 1.)

Certain diseases are carried in a person's genetic material (DNA) and can be passed from parent to child. Sometimes a child has a genetic disease when there has been no family history of the disease. This means there has been a mutation (i.e. an unexpected change in the DNA).

- There are over 4000 recognised genetic diseases
- A baby is born in the UK with a genetic disease or birth defect, on average, every 26 minutes.

Examples of genetically inherited diseases and conditions include:

- sickle cell anaemia
- haemophilia
- Huntington's chorea
- cystic fibrosis
- Down's syndrome.

The effect of these diseases on health and well-being varies from condition to condition, and person to person. A person suffering from a genetic disorder may suffer mild symptoms occasionally, or may be severely disabled with a short life expectancy.

There are a number of screening methods that can be used to detect a genetic disorder in an unborn baby (see pages 166–67).

- A pregnant woman will be offered a specialised blood test, which can indicate the risk of her baby having Down's syndrome.
- An ultrasound test, in which the tissues of the body are imaged using sound waves, can also indicate if there is a risk that the baby may have Downs Syndrome.
- If blood tests (see above) indicate that a woman has an increased risk of having a baby with Downs Syndrome, or if there is a family history of a genetic disorder, amniocentesis will be offered. This involves inserting a fine needle through the abdominal wall into the uterus and taking a sample of the amniotic fluid that surrounds the foetus. This sample contains cells from

the baby. The cells can be grown and the chromosomes can be examined for genetic disorders.

- Cells from the foetus can also be taken from the placenta, a technique known as **chorionic villus sampling (CVS)**.
- If a genetic disorder is detected, the mother will be offered a termination.

There are few examples of a genetic disease being cured. The cases that have been successful have involved children who suffer from a genetic disorder that affects their immune system. This means that they are often ill with infections and may not live to adulthood. It is possible to give these children a bone marrow transplant. If this is successful, they are cured and can then produce the cells needed to fight infection. It is hoped that, in the future, **gene therapy**, where people who lack the healthy gene can be given a replacement gene, will offer hope to individuals suffering from genetic disorders.

ACTIVITY

Choose an inherited disease or condition and find out about its:

- symptoms
- treatment.

If working in a group, each person can choose a different disease and then present their findings.

Illness and disease

(See also 'Illness and disease' on pages 22–3 in Chapter 1.)

When a person has an illness or disease, the physical effects are often obvious. However, it must be remembered that chronic disease may mean people have to face:

- time off work or school
- loss of employment
- loss of independence
- social isolation
- the possibility of death from the condition.

This means a person's intellectual, emotional and social health is likely to be affected. As mentioned in Chapter 1, a child's intellectual development may be affected if they miss important parts of their education. Emotional well-being of both the person with the disease and other family members can be affected as some diseases may cause shock and anxiety. The emotional effect will depend on the nature of the disease and the person affected. Illness can make people less resilient and so can lead to depression. Disease and illness can affect social-well being, as the person may be isolated from their friends and school or work colleagues.

Advice given to help people with chronic diseases (for example, cancer or diabetes) from sinking into depression includes:

- keep active, if appropriate (for example, people with lower back pain are now encouraged to return to work as soon as possible, and avoid bed rest)
- express emotions
- take control (for example, contribute to decisions about treatment)
- think positively (good support from family, friends and health professionals will help with this).

Diet

(See also *'Diet'* Chapter 1, page 23.)

A balanced diet

> 'You are what you eat.'
> 'A good diet is an important way of protecting health.'
> 'Eat yourself fit.'

These statements indicate the importance of diet to good health. A balanced diet has to contain the following:

- proteins
- carbohydrates
- fats
- fibre
- vitamins
- minerals
- water.

(See Figure 3.4.)

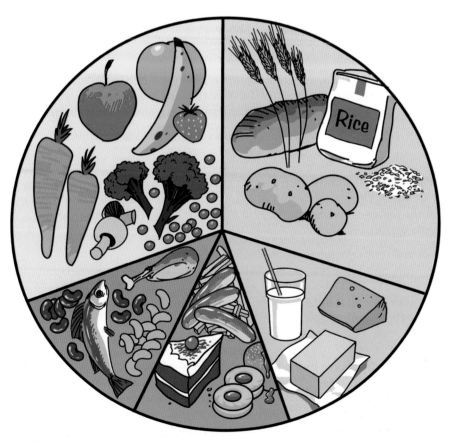

Figure 3.4 A balanced diet

ACTIVITY

Before you read further, which foods do you think are good sources of:

- protein
- carbohydrates
- fats
- energy?

(Check examples given in italics below.)

Carbohydrates

Carbohydrates are the most important source of energy in the diet. Because starchy foods release sugars more slowly and over a longer period of time into the blood, these foods are preferable to sugary foods.

Foods that are rich in carbohydrate are those which contain a lot of sugar, such as sweets and cakes, or those which contain a lot of starch, such as pasta, rice and bread.

Fats

Fats are a concentrated source of energy. They are necessary to provide us with fat-soluble vitamins, and they are an important part of cell membranes and some hormones. Plants tend to have liquid fats (oils) which are mainly unsaturated. Animal fats are solid at room temperature and are mainly saturated. (It is thought that an excess of saturated fat is particularly harmful to our health.)

Fat meat, and foods containing dairy products, animal fat or plant oils such as cakes and pastry, tend to be rich in fats.

Proteins

Proteins are required for growth and repair. They are needed to make enzymes (which control all the chemical reactions within the body), haemoglobin (which is the part of the red blood cells that carries oxygen), and cell membranes.

Meat, fish, cheese, eggs, nuts, grains and pulses are all good sources of protein.

Fibre

There is a type of carbohydrate, known as cellulose, which surrounds all plant cells. Cellulose cannot be broken down, so it remains undigested and is passed out in the faeces. This fibre helps food to keep moving though the gut and prevents constipation.

All fruit and vegetables are good sources of fibre.

Vitamins

Vitamins are essential in small amounts in the diet for maintaining good health. Table 3.1 gives some of their main uses and sources.

Minerals

We need 15 minerals (or inorganic salts) in our diet. Table 3.2 gives the uses and sources of some of these.

Water

Water is vital for health and is central to a balanced intake. A large proportion of food consists of water, and on top of this a person should aim to drink the equivalent of six to eight glasses of fluid a day.

Vitamin	Where from?	What for?	What happens if you don't get enough? (deficiency)
A	green leafy vegetables, liver	sight; bones/teeth	dry skin, skin sores; 'night blindness'; slow bone/tooth growth
D	made by skin using sunlight; also in oily fish, egg yolk, milk	bones	weak bones (rickets in children)
E	Nuts, seed oils, green leafy vegetables	wound healing, nerves	slow wound healing
K	made by bacteria in the gut; also in spinach, cauliflower, cabbage	blood clotting	slow blood clotting
B$_1$ (thiamin)	whole grain, eggs, pork, yeast	nerves	lack of energy; problems with digestion and nerves (beri-beri)
B2 (riboflavin)	yeast, meat, eggs, whole grain, peas, peanuts; small quantities produced by gut bacteria	release of energy from food	deficiency signs rarely seen
B$_3$ (niacin or nicotinamide)	yeast, meats, fish, whole grain, peas, beans	release of energy from food	pellagra (skin disease), diarrhoea
B$_{12}$	milk, eggs, cheese, meats	growth	anaemia
Folate (folic acid)	green leafy vegetables, made by gut bacteria	red/white blood cell production	anaemia; spine does not form correctly in foetus (spina bifida)
C (ascorbic acid)	citrus fruits, tomatoes, green vegetables	formation of connective tissue and wound healing	poor repair/growth (scurvy) including swollen gums, tooth loosening, fragile blood vessels; poor wound healing

Table 3.1 Vitamins

Mineral	Where from?	What for?	What happens if you don't get enough? (deficiency)
Calcium	Milk, egg yolk, shellfish, green leafy vegetables	Bones/teeth, blood clotting, muscle movement, growth	Weak bones (rickets in children)
Potassium	Widespread	Nerves, muscles	Problems with nervous system; heart attack

Table 3.2 Minerals

Mineral	Where from?	What for?	What happens if you don't get enough? (deficiency)
Sodium	Widespread, table salt	Salt/water balance of body	Problems with nervous system/ swelling of the brain
Magnesium	Beans, peanuts, bananas	Bones, muscles, nerves. Release of energy from food	Muscle weakness, fits, high blood pressure
Iron	Widespread but especially red meats, beans, fruits, nuts	Haemoglobin in red blood cells	Anaemia

Table 3.2 (continued)

Healthy eating – ten top tips

Because it is difficult for people to estimate whether they are having their recommended daily amounts of each type of nutrient in their diet, there are a number of useful guidelines worth remembering.

- Eat a wide variety of foods each day.
- Eat at least five 80 gram portions of fruit and vegetables every day.
- Eat lots of bread, other cereals or potatoes.
- Eat moderate amounts of lean meat, fish and alternatives.
- Eat moderate amounts of lower-fat milk and dairy foods (although children under two-years-old should not have reduced-fat milk).
- An average adult should drink about six to eight cups of liquid a day. (For example, water, fruit juice, skimmed or semi-skimmed milk, or low sugar soft drinks.)
- Avoid eating too much fat and fatty food, particularly saturated fats.
- Eat only small amounts of foods containing sugar.
- Use a minimum amount of salt in cooking and try not to add additional salt.
- Healthy food needn't be boring. A balanced diet can contain chips and chocolate – it's just a matter of getting the balance right.

An unbalanced, poor quality or inadequate diet

If a person's diet is not balanced, and has an excess or inadequate amount of particular nutrients, their health will suffer. In developing countries the most common causes of malnutrition are lack of protein and energy in the diet, but in developed countries unhealthy diets tend to include too much salt, sugar, and fatty foods which are linked to cancer, heart disease, stroke and tooth decay.

KEY TERM

Deficiency disease – condition caused by lack of a nutrient in the diet.

ACTIVITY

Look back at Tables 3.1 and 3.2 to check the deficiency diseases caused by the lack of vitamins and minerals.

Exercise

(See also 'Exercise' on pages 24–5 in Chapter 1.)

Why is exercise good for us?

Regular exercise can have a very positive effect on health at any age. Some of the physical effects of exercise are listed below, but it should also be remembered that any recreation undertaken in a group can also be good for a person's social health, and that exercising can lift feelings of mild depression, improve self-esteem, improve alertness and reduce stress.

The physical effects of exercise include:

- the heart becomes more efficient
- blood volume, red cells and haemoglobin increase
- arteries grow larger
- muscles used in breathing grow stronger
- lungs become more expandable and increase in volume
- coordination improves
- the muscles and tendons can be stretched more easily, thus increasing flexibility of joints
- muscles increase in strength
- it prevents obesity
- the immune system produces more white blood cells to help fight infection
- the chances of developing conditions like arthritis, high blood pressure, diabetes, stroke, osteoporosis (brittle bone disease) or heart disease later in life are reduced
- the effects of ageing are reduced.

The effect of exercise on the body depends on:

- the type of exercise and how vigorous it is
- the duration of the exercise
- the number of times a week the exercise is repeated
- how fit the person is already.

How much exercise do we need?

- To check that exercise is within safe limits, the maximum safe heart rate should be calculated by taking age away from 220. To improve fitness it is recommended that a person should exercise to produce a heart rate of 70%, the maximum safe heart rate for at least 20 minutes three times a week.
- Exercising below this heart rate can still help improve fitness, as long as it is carried out for longer; for example, 30 minutes of an activity which makes you slightly out of breath five times a week. The 30 minutes could be split into three 10-minute sessions in a day if preferred.
- People who are at risk of obesity need 45–60 minutes of exercise at least five times a week.
- The government recommends that children and young people get one hour of physical activity a day.

Exercise can be an activity that fits into daily life, such as a brisk walk to work or the shops, or it could be more structured exercise or sport, or a combination of both. The most important thing is that the person does something that they will enjoy, or at least put up with, so that they stick with it.

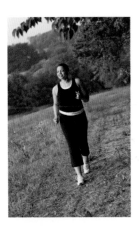

Figure 3.5 Brisk walking, swimming, cycling and dancing are all enjoyable ways to exercise

ACTIVITY

Look at the recommended amount of exercise above. If you are not already doing 5 × 30 min. each week, plan activities that you would enjoy doing and see how you could fit these into your week. (Note: Even short bursts of activity for 10 minutes or so add up to make a significant difference to your fitness.)

Alcohol

Some alcohol facts:

- There are an estimated 6500 deaths each year in England and Wales directly related to alcohol.
- Deaths from alcohol-related diseases have increased by more than a third in the past 10 years.
- One in 20 people are addicted to alcohol.
- About 38% of adult males drink above the recommended guidelines.
- Alcohol costs the NHS around £1.7 billion a year.
- Alcohol costs British industry an estimated £6.4 billion a year due to absenteeism and poor performance.
- Alcohol is a factor in 40% of domestic violence.

Figure 3.6 shows the long-term effects of alcohol on the body.

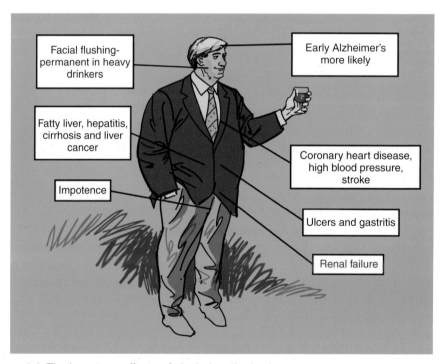

Figure 3.6 The long-term effects of alcohol on the body

Young people and alcohol

- In 2007 almost 5000 children under 18 were treated in hospital after drinking too much.
- More than half of teenagers drink by the age of 13.
- The average weekly amount of alcohol consumed by 11–15-year-olds has doubled in recent years (see Figure 3.7).
- Children between 10 and 15 who drink are twice as likely to commit a crime as those who do not.
- Regular teenage drinkers are responsible for a third of youth violence.
- Drinking means young people are far more likely to engage in risky behaviour; for example, unprotected sex.

Mean alcohol consumption (units) by 11–15-year-olds in last week, by gender: 1990–2006

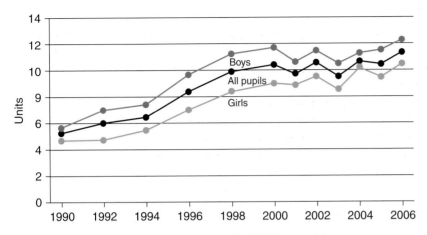

Figure 3.7 Average alcohol consumption by 11–15 year olds

To encourage parents to help their children drink responsibly, in early 2009 the government produced a table showing how much people can drink safely at different ages. It recommends that young people up to the age of 15 should avoid alcohol altogether (www.ah.gov.uk).

Pregnancy and alcohol

Alcohol can stop the normal development of the foetus. Babies born to mothers who drink large amounts of alcohol throughout the pregnancy may be born with foetal alcohol syndrome. These children have facial abnormalities, poor growth and severe mental and development problems. More moderate drinking may increase the risk of miscarriage, but many women continue to drink small amounts of alcohol throughout their pregnancy with no ill effects. Pregnant women are recommended to avoid alcohol if possible and, at the most, have no more than one or two alcoholic drinks a week. The same advice is given to women who are breastfeeding or trying to become pregnant.

Over 35s

Research has shown that around half of 35–54-year-olds rely on alcohol to unwind at the end of a stressful day. In 2008 a £10 million campaign was introduced to target middle-aged drinkers. It aimed to educate people about the number of units of alcohol in each drink, and to warn people who consumed two or three glasses of wine a night of the risks they faced. It emphasised the links between alcohol consumption and breast cancer, obesity and heart problems.

Older people and alcohol

- At least a third of older drinkers did not have a problem with alcohol until they reached the age of 60.
- Factors that can trigger heavy drinking include loneliness and isolation; bereavement; loss of skills, occupation or income.
- Older people are at greater risk of alcohol-related issues such as hypothermia, incontinence and depression.
- Older people may be affected more by alcohol and suffer a higher risk of accidents and falls. Alcohol use may contribute to memory loss or depression.
- Older people use the most prescription drugs, and alcohol can cause serious side effects when combined with many of these.

One of the most important things for drinkers to know is how the alcohol content of different drinks compare. Figure 3.8 shows drinks which contain roughly the same amount of alcohol. Each of these can be thought of as a unit.

Figure 3.9 shows the limits people should keep below to avoid damaging their health.

Figure 3.10 can be used to help a person keep a diary of their alcohol consumption for a typical week. At the end of the week, they can calculate the number of units consumed and compare this with the recommended limits. If the amount consumed is high, suitable opportunities for cutting down can be identified. (It is sometimes worth remembering HALT. This is to remind people that the occasions when there is the greatest temptation to drink too much are when someone is hungry, angry, lonely or tired.)

ACTIVITY

The following measures have been suggested to help limit the problems caused by excess drinking:

- the drink drive limits should be lowered
- more alcohol education should be provided for young people
- bottles and cans should be labelled with the number of units they contain
- supermarkets should be prevented from selling very cheap alcohol
- better services should be provided to people addicted to alcohol.

Discuss how useful you think each of these measures would be.

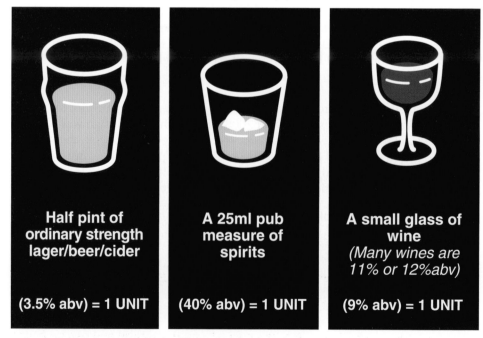

Figure 3.8 Drinks containing 1 unit of alcohol

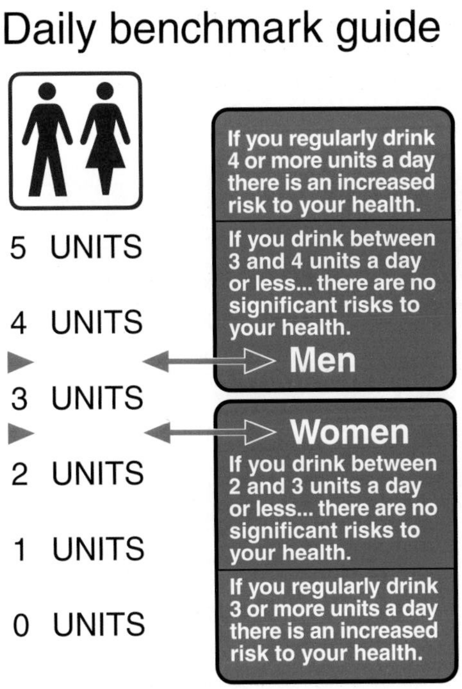

Daily benchmark guide
5 UNITS
4 UNITS
3 UNITS
2 UNITS
1 UNITS
0 UNITS
If you regularly drink 4 or more units a day there is an increased risk to your health.
If you drink between 3 and 4 units a day or less... there are no significant risks to your health.
Men
Women
If you drink between 2 and 3 units a day or less... there are no significant risks to your health.
If you regularly drink 3 or more units a day there is an increased risk to your health.

Figure 3.9 Limits to drinking to prevent damage to health

Drink Diary

	What?	*Where/When/Whom with?*	*Units*
Mon			
Tue			
Wed			
Thu			
Fri			
Sat			
Sun			
		TOTAL	

Figure 3.10 A drink diary

Smoking

Smoking is the biggest single cause of preventable disease and early death. There are five times more people killed by smoking than by road accidents, suicide, murder, AIDS and illegal drugs put together. Figure 3.11 shows that tobacco is easily the most dangerous substance in terms of deaths caused.

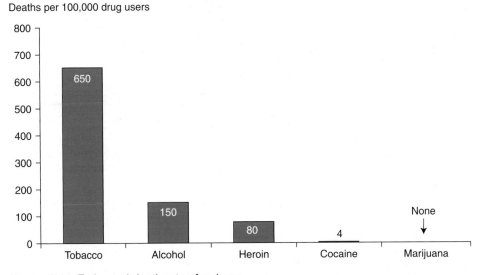

Deaths per 100,000 drug users
800
700
600
500
400
300
200
100
0
650
150
80
4
None
Tobacco
Alcohol
Heroin
Cocaine
Marijuana

Figure 3.11 Estimated death rates for drugs

Nicotine is the powerful drug in tobacco which causes physical and psychological addiction to smoking. It increases heart rate and blood pressure.

Tar is black and sticky and contains cancer-causing chemicals (carcinogens). Tar clogs up the lungs and the chemicals are gradually absorbed, causing irritation and damage.

Carbon monoxide is a harmful gas which makes blood less efficient at carrying oxygen to the brain and muscles.

The harmful effects of smoking are summarised in Figure 3.12.

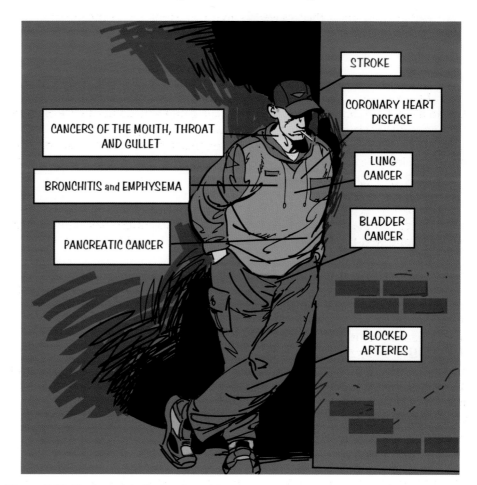

Figure 3.12 The harmful effects of smoking

Young people and smoking

The longer someone smokes, the greater their chance of serious health problems later on. Because nicotine is addictive, the earlier someone starts smoking, the harder it is to give up in later life.

Trying out new things and taking risks is part of growing up, and figures show that 60% of all 15-year-olds have smoked. Children are twice as likely to smoke if their parents are regular smokers.

Pregnancy, parenthood and smoking

A pregnant woman who smokes is:

- more likely to have an underweight baby
- twice as likely to have a premature baby
- a third more likely to have a stillborn baby
- more likely to have a miscarriage.

Children who have a parent who smokes are:

- at a higher risk of cot death
- a third more likely to suffer from glue ear, which causes partial deafness

- twice as likely to suffer from chest infections
- twice as likely to have asthma attacks.

17000 under-5s are in hospital because of their parent's smoking.

It is, therefore, important that, as well as giving up smoking for the duration of the pregnancy, parents should make every effort not to smoke in the company of their young children.

Older people and smoking

Studies have shown that smokers aged 65–74 years old are almost 10 times more likely to die of lung cancer than those of this age group who do not smoke. Because of the harmful effects of continuing to smoke, even in old age, it is important that elderly people consider trying to stop. However, this may be more difficult for them because the longer a person has smoked for, the stronger the addiction to nicotine.

Social, cultural and emotional factors

We have already seen in Chapter 1 that social, emotional and cultural factors have an effect on our personal development. These factors also have an effect on our health and well-being.

Family

Most of us belong to a family; we grow up as part of a family and when we get older we may have our own families. Research has shown that children whose parents smoke are more likely to smoke themselves. Children's diets are affected by the choices made by their parents. In a recent TV series which showed Jamie Oliver trying to develop healthy eating in schools, the mothers were pushing chips and other fast foods through the railings to their children at break time. The food that is eaten in a family may depend on the money available for food shopping. Cultural factors may also determine what types of foods are eaten by the family. Some religions ban the consumption of certain foods, like pork and animal products. Eating habits tend to be family based. Fewer homes have a separate dining room and many families eat while they look at TV, sitting on a sofa or easy chair. Because of shift work and weekend work, families are less likely to sit down to eat a meal together. Children may be expected to help themselves to food for their meals and fast foods and ready meals may be used instead of meals that are freshly prepared.

EXAMPLES

Example 1

Marie lives in rented accommodation. She has two children, Wayne who is 9 years old and Sharon who is aged 7. The children take packed lunches to school. A typical lunch box will include chocolate bars, crisps, a sandwich made with white sliced bread and a sugary drink.

After school the children look at TV, while they may have more crisps and a coke. In the evening they will have fish fingers and chips or sausages, while they look at a video.

Example 2

Charlotte and Ben live in the semi-detached house they are buying with a mortgage. They are both teachers but Charlotte works part time at the moment. They have three children Tom (8) Lisa (6) and Sam (4). The family are all vegetarians. The children have packed lunches. A typical lunch

(continued)

EXAMPLES – (continued)

box will include a humous sandwich made with wholemeal bread, two pieces of fruit, muesli bar, some sultanas and a drink (sugar free). They walk to school. After school they may go to music lessons (Tom and Lisa) or dancing class (Lisa and Sam). In the evening they have their supper round the table. They have pasta with tomato sauce followed by yoghurt and fruit. They have milk or fruit juice to drink.

ACTIVITY

Look at these two examples. Why do you think these two families eat different things? Is it just the amount of money that is available or are there other factors? Do you think there may be differences in what the family does in the following activities?

- seeing the dentist regularly
- the holidays they may have
- the after school activities they have
- the activities they do at weekends?

We can see from these two examples that families can affect our health and well-being throughout life. The family we are born into will influence what we do with our own families.

Friends

The friends we have throughout our lifetime can affect our health and well-being. While we are growing up our friends are very important to us. We may want to do the same things our friends do so that we feel we fit into the group we are part of. When we are young we may join football league teams, Guides or Rangers, or other clubs and classes simply because our friends belong to these. When we are teenagers, we may use alcohol, cigarettes and drugs because we want to fit in with our friends, who may also use these. We may do other activities that help our health and well-being such as belong to athletics clubs or play football or cricket and we may make friend there as well. When we are teenagers we may have a lot of pressure from our friends to do things that we know may not be good for our health and well-being – such as drinking too much or smoking. But it can be difficult if you belong to a group that does dangerous or illegal things. You want to fit in with your friends, but this may involve also doing dangerous or illegal things, like your friends.

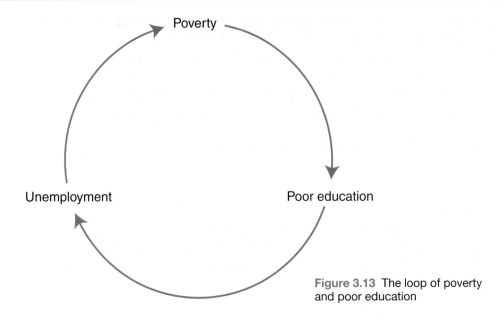

Figure 3.13 The loop of poverty and poor education

Educational experiences

(See also the section on *'Educational experiences'* on page 27 in Chapter 1.)

Education has been said to be 'the one way out of the dismal mixture of poverty, unemployment and crime' (see Figure 3.13).

Good education can improve health in a number of ways:

- It can inform pupils and students about health-related topics, such as diet and teenage pregnancy.
- It can improve a person's chances of employment and, therefore, make them less likely to suffer from poverty.
- It can improve a person's self-esteem; for example, research has shown that people with very low literacy are much more likely to be classified as depressed than those with good basic skills.

ACTIVITY

1. It has been suggested that schools should develop a 'healthy school' philosophy and, for example, put more emphasis on supplying healthy school meals, and reducing teenage pregnancies.

    In what ways do you think your school *helps* its students' health and well-being?

    In what ways do you think your school *could do more to help* its students' health and well-being?

2. It has been said that 'Teenage pregnancy is all too likely to be a cause as well as a symptom of poor education, unemployment and social exclusion. If a healthy school can keep a child from following her mother by getting pregnant at 17, she has a better chance of getting qualifications, getting a job, and breaking out of the loop.'

    (continued)

Employment/unemployment

Employment

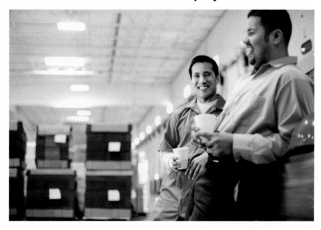

Figure 3.14 'Work can contribute positively to many aspects of health and well being'

Work can contribute positively to all aspects of health and wellbeing – physical, intellectual, emotional and social.

- Work can provide adequate financial resources, and prevent poverty (see 'Poverty' page 155, below).
- Working can also provide supportive relationships, and help to prevent social isolation (see Figure 3.14).
- People in employment are more likely to have better physical and mental health, live for longer and have higher self-esteem than those who are unemployed.

Unemployment

Ill-health can result from the stress and/or poverty caused by:

- unemployment
- job insecurity (the threat of being made unemployed)
- low wages.

There is a lot of evidence to show that people in employment have better physical and mental health than those who are unemployed. The following have all been found to be higher amongst the unemployed:

- death rates
- amount of long-term illness
- anxiety and depression
- risk of suicide
- heart disease
- stomach ulcers
- smoking
- obesity
- lack of self-esteem.

There are some groups of people who find it more difficult to get work than the general population. These include:

- people with mental health problems or physical disabilities
- homeless people
- people who have been in prison.

ACTIVITY

Health problems make it more difficult to find jobs, and, in turn, unemployment makes it difficult to stay healthy. This is described as the *downward spiral of health and employment*.

List the reasons you can think of why:

- health problems make it more difficult to find jobs
- unemployment makes it difficult to stay healthy.

Community involvement

As we have already seen in Chapter 1, getting involved in the community can help our personal development. It can also help our health and well-being. Local councils are developing many activities in response to the government's policy on Improving the Nation's Health. In one area the PCT and the local council are working together to help people improve their health. These are some of the examples they are developing:

- walking groups in the parks
- a healthy café in the park
- hiring out bicycles
- encouraging people to walk further by giving out a free pack containing pedometers
- a co-operative that sells fresh fruit and vegetables at low prices to people on a council estate
- running groups that encourage people to give up smoking
- chair-based exercises for people who cannot walk far
- free swimming at certain times
- advice on cooking cheaply using fresh produce.

Many of these schemes are staffed by volunteers who enjoy the activities and also benefit from improving their own health and well-being. The council has regular meetings in the different areas of the borough and people can influence decisions that are made about council spending. At a recent meeting the local residents wanted to reopen some disused toilets and to provide a café at the building as well. Volunteers will help staff the café. Many older people were worried about going out in the area when there was no toilet available. This is another example of community involvement influencing decisions made that can affect health and well-being.

Religion

As we have seen in Chapter 1, religion can help our personal development, but it can also help our health and well-being. Studies have shown that people who have a belief and pray for help to get them through an operation, may experience less pain and need less medication. Meditation is shown to have a positive effect on a person's health and well-being. If we belong to a religion that teaches us acceptance of life events and a belief in God's will, this may help to relieve stress that we might otherwise feel.

Gender

Men and women experience health and well-being differently. Women are more likely to talk about their problems to friends or to a professional. Men are more likely to put off seeking medical advice. Women are more likely to seek help for depression. Men would see admitting they have depression as a weakness. Women have certain experiences such as menstruation, childbirth and the menopause which men may find difficult to understand. Women are more likely to have tests to identify disease. Men are unwilling to take part in this.

ACTIVITY

It could be interesting if you asked five men and five women what health and well-being meant to them.

Do you think you would get different answers?

Ethnicity

Health and well-being can be seen differently in different ethnic communities. In parts of Africa a woman who is large (we would call obese) with large hips would be seen as more healthy than a thin woman. In parts of Africa depression is not seen as an illness and post-natal depression in not recognised. Ideas about body shape and function can vary across different ethnic groups; this is particularly the case with ideas about menstruation and childbirth. These differing views need to be taken into account by health and social care workers who look after these patients. In Western Society we are encouraged to be healthy, keep active and eat a balanced diet. Ethnic minorities may have differing ideas about health and well-being and this could cause conflict.

Sexual orientation

In personal development, sexuality is usually seen as having a heterosexual focus. This means that people are attracted to the opposite sex and this may impact on their health and well-being. Teenagers and men may go to the gym and try to present the male macho image that is in the media – with rippling muscles, a six-pack chest and an athletic lifestyle. Girls may try to work on their appearance so that they reflect the current image of heterosexual women. They may diet to achieve a model's figure. They may smoke and drink to boost their self-confidence and to appear older and more experienced than they are. These behaviours can be bad for their health and well-being. Girls and boys who are homosexual may feel uncomfortable with their heterosexual friends. 'Coming out' as gay can cause a great deal of stress for the young person and their families.

Culture

In chapter 1 we saw how culture can affect our personal development. It can also influence our health and well-being. Culture is related to our behaviour, diet, dress, language, and religious beliefs which all influence our lives. For example, some cultures have strict rues about the use of alcohol, marriage and other aspects of their lives. These strict rules may be difficult to follow in the UK. Arranged marriages still occur in some Asian families and girls who want to go out with English men and wear Western dress could be put under a great deal of stress because of the conflict with their families. Some customs, such as the practice of fasting in Ramadan could have a negative effect on young people, although people with medical conditions are exempt from observing strict fasting.

Relationship formation

During our lifetimes we expect to form close relationships with people outside our family. Some of these relationships can add to our sense of self-worth and encourage our personal development. However, some relationships can have negative effects on our health and well-being.

Look at the following examples of relationships and decide whether the relationship has a positive or negative impact on our health and well-being:

- John is married to Jane and he encourages her to go out with her friends.
- Abboo is concerned about his daughter meeting boys at her college, so he drives her to college and collects her at the end of the day.
- Ella has two close friends at college, Charlotte and Emma. Ella has a date with Mark. Emma tells Ella that if she goes out with Mark they won't be friends any more.
- Lisa is living with David. David has been diagnosed with depression. He sits at home all day and shouts at Lisa.
- Trevor and his mates are having a laugh in the pub. They have had a few pints and get into a fight. Trevor always seems to be the one who gets beaten up when this happens.

Relationships change as we get older and have new experiences. If we are in a long-term relationship with a partner, we need to adapt to changes as they happen whether it is illness, disability or the birth of a child. Many relationships can be helped through difficult times by support such as counselling. We know that emotional health is just as important as our physical health and that if relationships are damaging our health and well-being, we need to think very carefully about whether the relationship should continue.

Marriage

When two people decide to get married they make the vow to support each other in sickness and in health. However, marriage is not just the relationship between two people, but it also includes the birth families of husband and wife. We have all heard jokes about the 'interfering mother-in-law'. Sometimes the married couple's parents find it difficult to accept that their child is now committed to a partner. Marriage can be a good support. Jon, who recently married, says 'marriage makes me feel more settled and secure', as we know we are with someone who cares for us. However, married life can have its ups and downs with the arrival of children and stresses caused by money shortages, child care problems, illness, unemployment and other worries.

Divorce

Divorce is becoming more common in the UK. It is estimated that the average length of a marriage in the UK is 11 years (2008 figures). Divorce can affect our self-esteem and our personal development, but it can also have a negative impact on health and well-being. Men are more likely to be depressed after a divorce and use alcohol to cope with the situation. They may not be able to cook and clean and do other tasks that were done by their ex-wife. They may have limited access to any children from the marriage. Feminist studies showed that men are in better health when they are married, but women are in better health when they are single! Whatever the truth behind these studies, the health and well-being of men and women is affected by divorce.

Economic factors

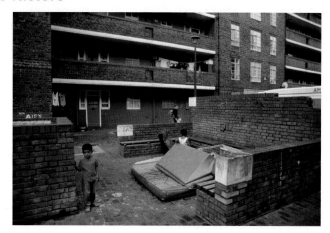

Figure 3.15 Economic factors have a significant effect on health and well-being

Income, wealth and material possessions

(See also '*Economic factors*' on pages 30–1, Chapter 1 and '*Poverty*' on page 155 below.)

An adequate income, level of wealth and a minimum level of material possessions is needed to ensure that a number of requirements for good health and well-being are met. Adequate economic factors will allow a person to have, for example:

- a healthy diet (see pages 137–140, above)
- satisfactory housing (see page 158, '*Housing conditions*', below)
- lower stress levels (see page 163, '*Stress*', below).
- access to adequate health care
- good personal hygiene.

There is evidence that, up to a certain point, increasing income, wealth and material possessions leads to increasing happiness, but at a certain level, a further increase has no effect.

Activities

1. As explained in Chapter 1, neither income, wealth or numerous material possessions can guarantee happiness. The New Economic Forum lists five actions that can be built into our day-to-day life, which research shows is important for the two main elements of well-being:
   i) Feeling good, for example, day to day, and overall happiness and satisfaction
   ii) Functioning well, for example, experiencing positive relationships, having control over one's life and having a sense of purpose.

The five actions are:

- **connect with people around you** (for example, family, friends, work or school colleagues and neighbours)
- **be active** (exercise)
- **take notice** (be aware of and curious about the world around you; be aware of your feelings; reflect on your experiences; enjoy the moment)
- **keep learning** (try something new; set yourself a challenge)
- **give** (do something for someone; volunteer your time; join a community group)

a) Discuss to what extent economic resources (income, wealth or material possessions) could help with each of these five actions.

b) List how a person could carry out each of the five actions without using income, wealth, or material possessions. (Suggested answers given)

2. Which of your material possessions do you consider to be absolutely necessary for your health and well-being? Compare your list with someone else. Do you agree with each other?

Employment status

(See also '*Employment/unemployment*' on page 27, Chapter 1; '*Employment status*' on page 32, Chapter 1; *and* '*Employment/unemployment*' on page 150, above.)

Employment status (i.e. whether a person is employed, or in a family where members are employed) will have a direct affect on income and therefore, as mentioned above, on health and well-being.

Social class and occupation

(See also '*Social class and occupation*' on page 33, Chapter 1.)

As mentioned in Chapter 1, one of the reasons for poorer health and well-being in people in lower social classes, is that they are more likely to live in poverty (see section below). This may be because of less regular employment and/or lower pay. This means they are likely to live in poorer housing conditions and to have a poorer diet. Both of these factors will have an adverse effect on health and well-being.

Poverty

There is a strong link between poverty and health, for example:

- The poorest people are more than twice as likely to die early as those who are better off.
- Around three children born to every 1000 parents who work in managerial and professional groups die before adulthood, compared with almost seven out of every 1000 parents from the lowest socio-economic groups.
- Women from poor socio-economic groups are more likely to have babies of low birth weight than women from higher socio-economic groups.

> **KEY TERM**
>
> Socio-economic group – the category people are put in depending on their social class, wealth and income and education.

Why poverty leads to poor health

There are a number of problems associated with poverty that adversely affect health.

- A person's income will affect their environment, education and housing.
- Smoking is more common amongst people in lower income groups; for example, unskilled workers are two or three times more likely to smoke than professionals.
- There are fewer primary care facilities available (for example, GP surgeries) in deprived areas.
- A family's inability to afford good quality food (food poverty) can cause long-term ill-health in children and affect development, behaviour and school performance.

What is poverty?

Families are considered to be living in poverty (i.e. below the poverty line) if their income is less than 60% of the average income. At 2008 values, the average income is £377, so the poverty line is set at £226.

Whether a person is considered to be below the poverty line depends on their situation. The rate for families is different from the rate for single people and couples with no children. Table 3.3 shows 2008 poverty lines.

	Weekly income (£)
Couple, two children aged 5 and 14	£346
Lone parent, two children aged 5 and 14	£271
Childless couple	£226
Single individual	£151

Table 3.3 '2008 poverty lines'

Certain groups face especially high risks of poverty.

Living in poverty in the UK:

- over a fifth of children (although the government aims to get rid of child poverty by 2020)
- about 23% of pensioners
- half of lone-parent families
- about 70% of families where the breadwinner is unemployed.

Relative poverty

Relative poverty means being poor in a rich society, and it is thought that this has a worse effect on health than being poor in a poor society. Societies with small differences between incomes have lower death rates than societies with large differences between incomes. A report in 2008 showed that in the UK, the gap between the people with the lowest incomes (mainly pensioners, children and women) and the people with the highest incomes is growing. The richest fifth of households share 43% of the national income, but the poorest fifth of households only share 7% of the national income.

Physical environment factors

Pollution

Pollution of the environment can have a significant effect on our health and well-being. Aspects of pollution that can have an impact on health are:

- air pollution
- water pollution.

Air pollution

In the long term, air quality has improved and most of the time, air pollution levels are low. However, research suggests that poor air quality is responsible for more than 32 000 deaths in the UK each year.

Table 3.4 shows the five main pollutants in the air and their effects on health. These come from sources such as car exhaust fumes, power stations, domestic fires, industry and cigarette smoke.

Air pollution can be harmful for people, particularly the elderly, with lung diseases, such as asthma, bronchitis and emphysema and heart disease.

If your health is good, it will be unlikely that you will be affected by air pollution. However, at very high levels of pollution, people may feel eye irritation, cough and feel it hurts when breathing deeply.

KEY TERMS

Asthma – a disease in which there is narrowing of the airways, leading to wheezing, coughing, tightness of the chest and shortness of breath.

Bronchitis – a disease in which the small airways are blocked and damaged, leading to a severe cough producing large quantities of phlegm (a mix of mucus, bacteria and white blood cells).

Emphysema – a disease in which there is breakdown of air sacs in the lungs, leading to wheezing and shortness of breath.

Pollutant	Health effects at very high levels
Nitrogen dioxide Sulphur dioxide Ozone	These gases irritate the airways of the lungs, increasing the symptoms of those suffering from lung diseases.
Particles	Fine particles can be carried deep into the lungs where they can cause inflammation and a worsening of heart and lung diseases.
Carbon monoxide	This gas prevents the normal transport of oxygen by the blood. This can lead to a reduction in the supply of oxygen to the heart, particularly in people suffering from heart disease.

Source: From page 10 'Air pollution: what it means for your health; the public information service' produced by Defra

Table 3.4 Health effects of five most common pollutants

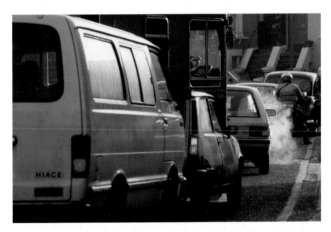

Figure 3.16 Traffic is one of the main sources of air pollution

ACTIVITY

1. One way to cut down on the air pollution is to reduce our use of cars (Figure 3.16).
   (i) If your family has a car, can you think of ways in which you could reduce your number of car journeys?
   (ii) Can you think of ways of encouraging other people to reduce their dependence on cars? Are there any examples in your local area?
2. You can find out about air pollution levels in your area from the website www.airquality.co.uk.

Water pollution

Humans need water for a variety of uses. It must be clear and not contaminated with pollutants, in order to prevent infectious diseases and poisoning. Toxic (poisonous) chemicals, industrial, agricultural and domestic waste are common pollutants of water. Purification is carried out on water before it is used, but although the treatment can remove organic waste and some bacterial contamination, it cannot cope with heavy chemical pollution. Examples of chemical pollutants in water include the following:

- **Heavy metals** from industry can go into lakes and rivers. These can be taken in by fish and then pass to humans. They can slow development, and cause cancer and birth defects.
- **Nitrates** enter water from fertilisers which are washed out of soil.
- **Microbes, such as bacteria** can cause disease. This is a major problem in developing countries.

The Environment Agency is responsible for maintaining or improving the quality of water in lakes, rivers and the sea in England and Wales.

The Drinking Water Inspectorate (DWI) is responsible for the quality of water in our taps. **Local Authority Environmental Health Departments** have local responsibility and often carry out random sampling.

Noise

Environmental noise is unwanted or harmful outdoor sound created by human activities. Noise can have a negative impact on quality of life, so it is bound to affect health and well-being. Examples include noise from transport, such as road, rail and air traffic and industry. Because it can be a health hazard, noise is considered as a form of pollution.

- Sounds above 90 dB (decibels) can damage hearing. If exposure is over a long period, this damage can be permanent.
- Noise causes the production of stress hormones and long-term exposure can possibly cause heart disease and even heart attacks.
- Noise can disturb people's sleep patterns, which can have consequences for their health.
- Research suggests that noise can have an adverse effect on mental health.

ACTIVITY

Noise maps were produced in 2006–7 by the government. You can visit the noise mapping website (www.noisemapping.defra.gov.uk) to find out about noise levels in the area where you live. They show that there are very few tranquil areas remaining in Britain. With forecasts of huge traffic increases in the next 20 years, noise levels are set to increase further.

KEY TERM

Social exclusion – when an individual is prevented from taking part in any of the key economic, social and political activities in the society in which they live.

Housing conditions

It is difficult to know to what extent poor housing affects health. This is because people who live in unhealthy homes usually suffer from other forms of disadvantage, such as poor diet, unemployment or poor education.

The groups most affected by inadequate housing are:

- The elderly
- Young children and babies
- Long term ill
- Disabled people
- Households with many people.

Shelter, a housing charity says, *'Children trapped in bad housing have the odds stacked against them. Without the security of a decent home, they lose out on vital schooling, endure mental and physical ill-health and fall into a cycle of social exclusion and poverty.'*

Characteristics of poor housing that have a direct effect on health

- **Faulty design** may contribute to fires and falls in the home. Most house fires occur in poor and inadequate housing. Children from the lowest social class are 40 times more likely to die in a house fire than people from the highest social class.
- **Inadequate lighting** can be linked to falls.
- **Defective and inadequate electrical wiring** increases the risk of injury from electric shocks, house fires, and tripping over trailing wires.
- **Damp** is related to the growth of moulds and mites, and thus linked to respiratory diseases such as asthma and bronchitis. It can also make conditions such as arthritis and rheumatism worse and affect mental health, for example depression.
- **Inadequate heating** may lead to hypothermia, particularly in the elderly. A cold home also makes respiratory illnesses, cardiovascular conditions and mental health conditions, such as depression, more likely. Arthritis and rheumatism may be worse. Old people are at a higher risk of accidents and falls in a cold home. The poorest people usually live in **badly insulated** homes, which are the most expensive to heat. The term **'fuel poverty'** is used to describe a situation where a person struggles to afford to heat their home.
- **Defective gas appliances or a coal fire** gives the risk of carbon monoxide poisoning, explosions or fires from blocked chimneys or flues.
- **Poor sanitation**, for example the shared washing facilities in bedsits and bed-and-breakfast hostels, can lead to the spread of disease.
- **Inadequate food storage and cooking facilities** increase the incidence of food poisoning and make a poor diet more likely.
- **Overcrowding** means some diseases that are caused by viruses or bacteria spread more easily. The housing charity, Shelter, say that children living in overcrowded housing are 10 times more likely to have meningitis.

KEY TERMS
Respiratory diseases – conditions that affect breathing, such as asthma and bronchitis (see key terms on page 156).
Cardiovascular diseases – conditions that affect the heart and circulation (see key terms on page 176 below).

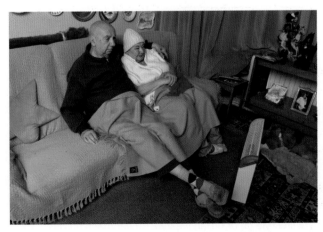

Figure 3.17 Inadequate housing can have a direct effect on health

CASE STUDY – Sally

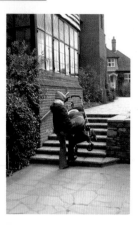

Figure 3.18

Sally lives with her child, Sam, in bed-and-breakfast accommodation. They have one room and share a kitchen, toilet and bathroom with two other families. Their room is on the second floor which makes life difficult, as Sam is still in a pushchair. In their room there is a problem with damp in the winter, and this is made worse because Sally has to dry their clothes on a radiator. There are no nearby shops, so she often has to rely on fish and chips from the mobile food van that visits. When she leaves food in the shared fridge it often disappears, so she keeps most of their food in the bottom of her wardrobe. Sally gets fed up with all the rules: children aren't allowed to play in the corridor; there is no hot water after 10 pm; the kitchen is locked at 9 pm; no visitors are allowed. Since they have lived there, Sam has suffered from asthma, Sally occasionally has a bad back, and they both sometimes have diarrhoea. Recently Sally has been feeling depressed.

ACTIVITY

Read the account above of a young mother's living conditions. Write a list of the health problems she and her young child have, and for each suggest how these may have been caused by aspects of their housing.

Rural/urban lifestyles

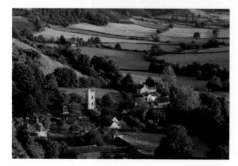 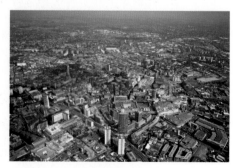

Figure 3.19 A rural lifestyle (a) or urban lifestyle (b) can have an affect on health and well being

Table 3.5 shows some of the advantages of living in rural or urban areas.

Advantages of living in a rural community	Advantages of living in an urban community
Lower crime rate	Better public transport
Better air quality and less noise pollution	Better access to services (e.g. schools, health centres and hospitals)
Natural/agricultural environment	More leisure facilities
Close-knit communities	Better employment opportunities
On average, less deprivation (although there are a number of rural areas where there poverty is a serious issue)	More social opportunities

Table 3.5 Some of the advantages of living in rural or urban areas

In rural areas there tends to be a higher standard of health and well-being than in urban areas. This is shown by a number of standard measures of health, such as life expectancy and infant mortality. Research suggests that the main reason for this is that, on average, rural populations tend to be less deprived than urban populations.

In 2008, the Office for National Statistics released figures that showed significant differences between rural and urban areas in terms of health and well-being. Death rates were found to be higher in urban areas and lowest in the least densely-populated rural areas. This can be explained partly by differences in deprivation between the different areas. However, even when the figures are adjusted to take deprivation into account, there is still a significant difference.

- Death rate for males in England is 15% lower in rural areas than it is in urban areas (3% difference if deprivation taken into consideration).
- Death rate for females in England is 9% lower in rural areas than it is in urban areas (no difference if deprivation taken into consideration).
- Death rate for males in Wales is 10% lower in rural areas than it is in urban areas (5% difference if deprivation taken into consideration).
- Death rate for females in Wales is 8% lower in rural areas than it is in urban areas (4% difference if deprivation taken into consideration).

The death rates also differ between urban and rural areas for certain diseases, for example:

- Death rates from lung cancer in rural areas of England in 2002–4, were 10% lower for males and 11% lower for females than in urban areas after allowing for deprivation. Research suggests that this may be because there is a lower rate of smoking and better air quality (see section on '*Pollution*', above) in rural areas.
- Death rates from accidents in rural areas of England in 2002–4, were 23% *higher* for males and 12% higher for females than in urban areas after allowing for deprivation. Research suggests that this may be because road traffic collisions are more likely to be fatal in rural areas, even though they are more common in urban areas.
- Death rates from suicide in rural areas of England in 2002–4, were 11% *higher* for males than in urban areas after allowing for deprivation. (There was no difference for females.)

Those living in rural areas make less use of health services and have a more positive view of their own health. The level of mental health problems is lower in rural areas. However, there may be particular problems in rural areas, such as people being reluctant to seek help for health problems. In recognition of this, some rural organisations have been set up to help people, for example the Rural Stress Information Network and Farm Crisis Network. These provide confidential support at a local level. If an organisation covers a rural catchment area, the government encourages them to 'rural proof' policies or services, which means they should take account of the needs of rural communities. The aim of rural proofing is to help overcome the disadvantages that people living in rural areas may experience in their access to services.

ACTIVITY

Read the two case studies below and list the problems faced by Sarah, who lives in a rural area, and Ahmed, who lives in an urban area. What do you think may be the advantages their rural or urban lifestyles bring?

CASE STUDY – Sarah

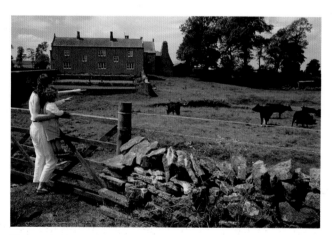

Figure 3.20

Sarah, 20, lives in a small village in Devon with her 2-year-old son, Jack. She takes him to a parent and toddlers group twice a week, which they both enjoy. For minor health problems and developmental checks, they can go to the health centre in the village. However, at the start of her pregnancy, Sarah says she avoided going to there 'because I didn't want everyone to know my business'. Sarah doesn't drive, and the buses to the nearest city, which is fifteen miles away, are infrequent. Last year, when she had to attend a series of hospital appointments she had to rely on a voluntary organisation, Morecare, to take her. She says she would like to do a part-time course or job, but there is nothing available locally.

CASE STUDY – Ahmed

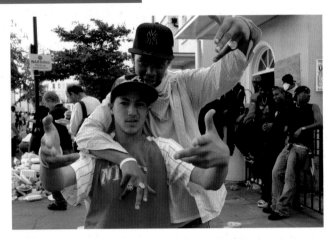

Figure 3.21

Ahmed, 13, lives with his parents in an urban area on the outskirts of a city. His school is about a mile from his house, and he travels there by bus. At the weekend he sometimes goes to the cinema with his friends and his father drives him there because, since he read a story in the local newspaper about a teenager being mugged, he worries about Ahmed being out in the evening. His parents complain about the noise of planes from the nearby airport, but Ahmed says he only notices this occasionally.

ACTIVITY

Debate the motion 'A rural lifestyle is healthier than an urban lifestyle'.

Psychological factors

Stress

If there is a change in a person's life that they find difficult to cope with, we say they are suffering from stress.

Stress and performance

If a person is under excessive stress, they will perform a task poorly. However, stress should not always be thought of as entirely negative. If a person is completely lacking stress, to the point at which they are bored, there will also be a decline in their ability to perform a task (Figure 3.22). This means that for each person there will be an optimum level of stress that will help them perform to the best of their ability.

Stress and health

Stress and how we manage our stress levels is linked directly to our health. A constant high level of stress will lead to physical, emotional and intellectual ill-health.

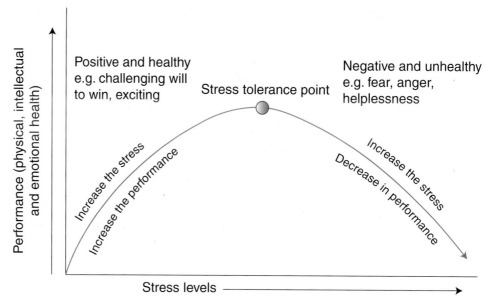

Figure 3.22 The relationship between amount of stress and the ability to perform a task

When a person is under stress, the hormone **adrenaline** is produced. This hormone prepares you for what is known as the '**fight or flight**' reaction. Some of the effects of adrenaline include:

- an increased heart rate
- less blood flowing through the skin, which may make a person appear pale
- less blood flowing around the gut, which leads to the feeling of 'butterflies'
- increased sweating.

If the stress continues, eventually the person will become ill. In 2006–7 13.8 million working days were lost because of stress-related illnesses, and it is estimated that these cost £7 billion per year in sick pay, lost production and health service provision.

Stress has various effects on a person's health. For example:

- **physical health problems**, such as stomach ulcers, heart attacks, skin disorders such as eczema and psoriasis, ME
- **emotional effects**, such as anxiety, insomnia and depression
- **behavioural effects**, such as increased smoking or consumption of alcohol.

Table 3.6 shows many of the short-term and long-term symptoms of stress.

Coping with stress

Methods of coping with stressful situations may be either beneficial to a person's health or harmful to their health. For example, if you have an examination on a topic you find difficult, you may choose any of the following methods to help you cope, some of which are beneficial and some of which are harmful.

Methods of coping which are beneficial to health

- **Changing work patterns** – for example, you could draw up a revision timetable which allows you to spend an hour going through the work each evening with a friend.
- **Exercise** – for example, you could make time to go for an early morning swim.
- **The use of relaxation techniques** – for example, you could attend a yoga class.
- **A healthy diet** – you should make time to enjoy healthy, well-balanced meals.

Behavioural short-term	Physical short-term	Emotional short-term
Over indulgence in smoking, alcohol or drugs Accidents Impulsive, emotional behaviour Poor relationships with others at home and at work Poor work performance Emotional withdrawal	Headaches Back aches Sleeping badly Indigestion Nausea Dizziness Excessive sweating Trembling	Tiredness Anxiety Boredom Irritability Depression Inability to concentrate Apathy
Behavioural long-term	**Physical long-term**	**Emotional long-term**
Marital and family breakdown Social isolation	Heart disease High blood pressure Ulcers Poor general health	Insomnia Chronic depression and anxiety

(From 'Stress at work' Health and safety leaflet published by Unison)

Table 3.6 Symptoms of stress

- **An increase in leisure time** – for example, you could spend time at the weekend relaxing with friends.
- **Rest** – you should make sure you have at least 6–8 hours sleep a night.

Methods of coping which are harmful to health

- Increased use of tobacco, alcohol, tranquillisers, sleeping pills or illegal drugs.
- Long hours of studying, causing lack of sleep.

Relationships within the family, and with friends and partners

Read the section above in this chapter on *'Relationship formation'* (page 153) to remind yourself of both the negative and positive effects that relationships with family, friends and partners can have on an individual's health and well-being.

Health monitoring and illness prevention services

The increase in health monitoring and illness prevention services has led to an improvement in the health of the population. Health monitoring includes the use of screening, and illness prevention services including vaccination. These are described below.

Screening

A screening test is a simple test carried out on a large number of apparently healthy people to identifying those who probably have a certain disease, or are at risk of developing a disease.

Screening programmes can be:

- for specific groups, for example for pregnant women, newborn babies, children, women, men, or older people
- for particular diseases, for example breast cancer.

Advantages of screening

- Individuals can make more informed choices about their health.
- Treatment can be given before a person shows signs of ill-health.

- Screening can reduce the risk of a person developing a condition or its complications.
- Screening has the potential to save lives or improve the quality of life.

Disadvantages of screening

- Screening cannot guarantee protection against a disease.
- A positive result (i.e. disease present) may lead to increased stress.
- People will occasionally be told they have the condition when they don't (false positive results).
- People will occasionally be told they don't have the condition when they do (false negative results).
- Worry that confidentiality of results cannot be guaranteed.
- Worry that there may be discrimination by insurance companies or employers against people known to have a disease, or who are at risk of developing a disease.

Examples of screening programmes

i) Antenatal screening for the baby

Antenatal screening is a way of checking whether an unborn baby (foetus) could develop, or has developed an abnormality during pregnancy. Screening is not the same as diagnosis. It indicates how *likely* a baby is to develop certain conditions. If the risk is found to be high, the mother may be offered further tests that will diagnose more accurately if the condition is present; for example, if a screening test shows that there is a 1 in 250 chance that the baby will have Downs Syndrome, the mother will be offered a diagnostic test. Examples of diagnostic tests include amniocentesis and chorionic villus sampling (CVS). (See page 135, above, *'Genetic inheritance'*.)

If after screening, the further diagnostic tests show that the foetus has an abnormality:

- the mother could choose to have an abortion
- the family could prepare psychologically and practically for a baby with abnormalities
- health professionals could prepare to start treatment immediately after the birth.

In the UK all women are offered (but do not have to accept) the following tests for their unborn baby:

- Downs Syndrome
- Sickle cell disease (an inherited blood disease)
- Thalassaemia (an inherited blood disease)
- Spina bifida (spine not correctly formed).

A combination of techniques is used:

- Blood tests Blood is taken from the mother between weeks 11 and 20 of the pregnancy. The levels of proteins and hormones indicate the chance of a baby having Downs Syndrome or spina bifida.
- Ultrasound scanning This is carried out at 18–20 weeks of the pregnancy.

ii) Antenatal screening for the mother

A woman will have check-ups through the pregnancy to test for conditions that could be harmful to the baby. The diseases looked for are:

- Anaemia
- HIV
- Hepatitis B
- Rubella (German measles)
- Urinary tract infections

KEY TERMS

Antenatal screening test – test to identify women and their babies who may be at slightly higher risk of having complications in pregnancy.

Diagnostic test – test that confirms if a foetus has an abnormality.

- Syphilis
- High blood pressure
- Diabetes.

iii) Neonatal screening

All babies are examined as soon as possible after the birth and again at six weeks. Screening tests are carried out to check for specific disorders that can be successfully treated if detected early enough. They include tests for:

- Anatomical abnormalities
- dislocation of the hip
- heart disease
- cataracts
- undescended testes.

A heel prick blood sample is taken from the baby in the first few days after birth to test for:

- phenylketonuria and MCADD (conditions that cause severe disability but, once detected, can be treated simply with diet)
- thyroid function
- cystic fibrosis (causes problems in the lungs and digestive tract)
- sickle cell anaemia (an inherited blood condition found in some ethnic groups).

Hearing screening is offered to all babies in the UK by 4–5 weeks old.

iv) Childhood screening

Over the first few years of a child's life a number of other conditions will be checked for; for example, tests will be made for:

- cataracts
- heart defects
- normal hearing
- normal growth.

v) Screening programmes for adults

There are nationally coordinated screening programmes for:

- Breast cancer
- Abnormalities that could lead to cervical cancer
- Bowel cancer.

Vaccination (Immunisation)

When bacteria or viruses enter the body, the immune system makes antibodies to destroy them. These antibodies stick to the invader and destroy it.

When a vaccine is given it makes the body produce antibodies but does not actually cause the disease. This means that later, when the person comes into contact with the disease, their immune system will respond rapidly and the bacteria and viruses will quickly be killed (see Figure 3.23).

There are a number of different types of vaccine:

- Live vaccine – a very weak preparation of a living, disease-causing bacteria or virus
- Preparation of dead disease-causing bacteria or viruses

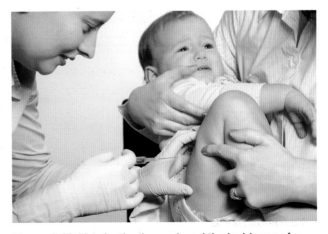

Figure 3.23 Vaccination has reduced the incidence of many diseases

- Extracts of toxins – this is a preparation of poisonous substances from the bacteria, which has been made harmless.

Table 3.7 shows the diseases that are commonly vaccinated for.

Disease	Description	Vaccination
Diptheria	Starts with a sore throat but can rapidly get worse, leading to severe breathing difficulties. Can also damage heart and nervous system	DTaP
Tetanus	Bacteria from soil gets into body through cuts and causes muscle stiffness	DTaP
Pertussis (whooping cough)	Severe whooping cough which can last for months and cause breathing problems and even deaths	DTaP
Polio	Virus that attacks nervous system and can paralyse muscles permanently. Can be fatal if it attacks muscles in the chest or used for swallowing	IPV
Hib meningitis	Caused by a lethal bacterium that causes meningitis and swelling of the throat	Hib
Pneumococcal infection	Pneumococcal bacteria cause pneumonia, septicaemia (blood poisoning), meningitis and ear infections	PCV
Meningitis C	Before the vaccine, this was the most common killer in the 1–5 age group. Bacteria cause brain and blood infection	Men C
Measles	Highly contagious virus that causes high temperature and rash. In 60% of cases there are complications such as chest infections, fits and brain damage. Can kill	MMR
Mumps	Virus causes swelling of salivary glands	MMR
Rubella (German measles)	Rash caused by virus. In pregnant women may cause severe damage to the unborn baby (e.g. blindness, brain damage)	MMR
Tuberculosis (TB)	Bacteria that attacks lungs, but can affect rest of body	BCG
Hepatitis B	Virus that damages the liver	Hep B
Cervical cancer	Human papilloma virus can cause cancer of the cervix (neck of the womb)	HPV

Table 3.7 Diseases for which vaccines are available

Vaccination programmes in the UK

Table 3.8 shows the routine immunisation programme in the UK in 2008.

Age	Diseases vaccinated against
Routine childhood immunisation	
2 months	Diptheria, tetanus, pertussis (whooping cough), polio, Hib, Pneumococcal infection
3 months	Diptheria, tetanus, pertussis (whooping cough), polio, Hib, meningitis C
4 months	Diptheria, tetanus, pertussis (whooping cough), polio, Hib, meningitis C, Pneumococcal infection
12 months	Hib, meningitis C
13 months	Measles, mumps, rubella, Pneumococcal infection
3 years and 4 months	Diptheria, tetanus, pertussis (whooping cough), polio, measles, mumps, rubella
13–18 years old	Diptheria, tetanus, polio, and for girls only human papilloma virus (HPV)
Non-routine immunisations	
Birth (babies more likely than the general population to come into contact with TB; if not, given at secondary school)	Tuberculosis (TB)
Birth (if mother is hepatitis B positive)	Hepatitis B

Table 3.8 Routine immunisation programme in the UK in 2008

Most diseases require more than one dose of a vaccine to give adequate protection. These are known as 'boosters'.

- HPV vaccination was introduced to the national immunisation programme in September 2008, for girls 12–13 across the UK to prevent them developing cervical cancer. In Autumn 2009, there will be a two-year catch up campaign to vaccinate all girls up to 18 years of age. It will be many years before the HPV vaccination programme has an effect on the number of cases of cervical cancer, so women are advised that they should still accept their invitations for cervical screening.
- It is hoped that in the future a vaccine for meningitis B will be included in the immunisation programme. There are roughly 1200 cases of this disease in the UK each year, of which 10% result in death.

Assessing the risk of immunisation

In recent years, some parents became so concerned about possible side effects of immunisation, that they have not had their children vaccinated. In some areas of the country, more than a third of 5-year-olds have not been properly immunised against measles, mumps and rubella. There is now concern that there could be outbreaks of measles, a very infectious viral disease that spreads in droplets in the air when people cough or sneeze. In some children there can be severe complications which can result in death. The Health Protection Agency (HPA) recommends that if a child has missed one, or both MMR doses, parents should contact their GP to arrange vaccination.

When assessing the risk of immunisation, parents need to compare how likely it is that there will be complications if a child *is* vaccinated, compared with how likely it is that there will be complications if a child is *not* vaccinated.

- With the MMR vaccine there is a risk of 1 in 1000 of febrile convulsions (fits).
- If a child catches measles, the risk of convulsions is 1 in 200.

Indicators of physical health

Measurements can be made to assess the state of an individual's health and well-being. Examples include:

- blood pressure
- peak flow
- body mass index
- hip/waist ratio measures
- body fat composition
- cholesterol levels
- blood glucose tests
- liver function tests
- resting pulse and recovery after exercise.

A person's age, sex and lifestyle must be taken into account when interpreting these measurements.

Blood pressure

The pressure at which blood flows through the circulatory system can be used as an indicator of health. It is measured using a sphygmomanometer (or sphygmo for short). Traditionally, a mercury column sphygmomanometer was used for measuring blood pressure, so we still use the unit mmHg. However, now an electronic model is used (see Figure 3.24). A cuff is inflated around the upper arm. The high pressure squeezes the brachial artery which stops the blood flow to the lower arm. The cuff is then slowly deflated and, as the blood flow resumes, the sounds are detected by the microphone that is built into the cuff. Measurements are read from a gauge or digital display. Some models provide a reading of pulse as well.

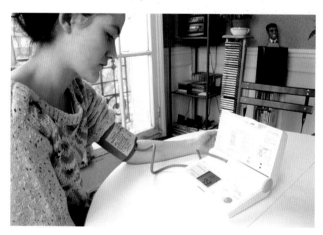

Figure 3.24 Measuring blood pressure using a sphygmomanometer

Blood pressure is recorded as two numbers – the systolic over diastolic pressure.

- The systolic pressure is the pressure when the heart is contracting and is therefore the higher value.
- The diastolic pressure is the pressure when the heart is relaxing and is therefore the lower value.
- 120/80 mmHg is a normal reading, but there is great variation between individuals. Blood pressure increases with age.
- A person who suffers from hypotension has a low blood pressure.
- A person who suffers from hypertension has a high blood pressure. A blood pressure of more than 140 systolic and 90 diastolic is considered abnormal.

ACTIVITY

If you have access to a digital blood pressure monitor, have a go at measuring your blood pressure, following the instructions provided.

Safety precautions:

- *Never use a sphygmomanometer unsupervised.*
- *Do not over inflate the cuff or leave in place for longer than necessary.*
- *If you get an unusual reading, don't worry as unreliable figures may be obtained in a classroom situation.*
- *It is recommended that people who use a monitor to check their own blood pressure, should check any unusual readings with a health professional.*

Peak flow

Peak flow is a measure of how fast you can blow air out of your lungs. It can be measured with a peak flow meter (see Figure 3.25).

When you blow into a peak flow meter it measures the speed of air passing through the meter. This figure is given in cubic decimetres (dm^3, i.e. litres) per minute. Peak flow readings vary according to sex, age, height and even the time of day the measurement is taken.

- Peak flow readings are usually higher in men than women.
- The highest peak flow usually occurs between the ages of 30 to 40 years.
- The taller a person is, the higher their peak flow is likely to be.
- Peak flow is often higher in the morning than in the evening.

Peak flow measurements are often used to diagnose and monitor the severity of asthma. People with asthma have narrowed airways taking air to the lungs, which reduce the flow of air. This means that asthma sufferers will have a low peak flow reading and the more severe their asthma, the lower their reading. Asthma sufferers will have a peak flow reading of 200–400 dm^3/min, compared with a normal value of 400–600 dm^3/min. Because peak flow may vary a lot from time to time, a one-off reading at a surgery may not give a doctor or nurse sufficient information. The asthma sufferer will, therefore, be asked to take their own readings morning and evening over a period of time and plot them on a chart (see Figure 3.26).

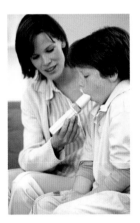

Figure 3.25 A peak flow meter

Body Mass Index (BMI)

A person's weight can be an important guide to their physical health. If someone is very overweight or underweight, it is obviously cause for concern about their physical health. However, as the example below shows, a measurement of weight alone will not give sufficient information to allow conclusions to be reached about physical fitness.

ACTIVITY

Paul is an 18-year-old student who weighs 77 kg. Can you make any comments on the state of his physical health?

What other piece of information would be most useful to help you form an opinion?

To allow any conclusions to be drawn about physical health from the weight of a person, we obviously need to have an idea of their height too. In the example

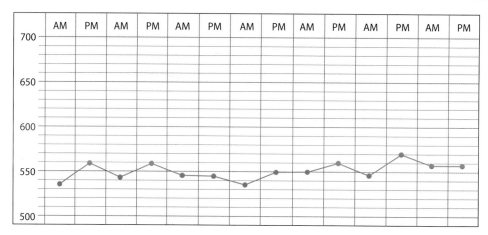

1. Peak flow chart of a person without asthma or a person whose asthma is well controlled

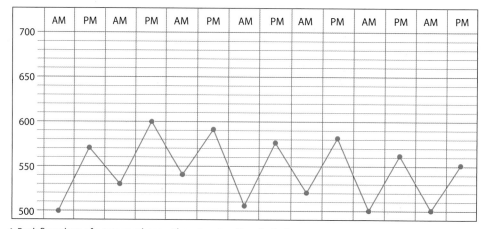

1. Peak flow chart of a person whose asthma is not well controlled

Figure 3.26 Peak flow charts

above, you would have formed a different opinion of Paul's physical health if you had been told that he was 1.83 m or 1.60 m.

Height should be measured as shown in Figure 3.27.

ACTIVITY

Figure 3.28 shows the relationship between weights and heights.

1. Take a straight line across from your height and a line up from your weight. (When you weigh yourself, take 2 kg off to allow for your clothes.) Check which category you fit into. Does this mean you need to alter your diet/exercise regime? If so, how?

Body mass index is a measure that takes into account both height and weight. It can, therefore, be used to indicate whether a person's weight is healthy for their height.

Body mass index (BMI) is given by the equation:

$$BMI = \frac{mass\ (kg)}{height\ (m)^2}$$

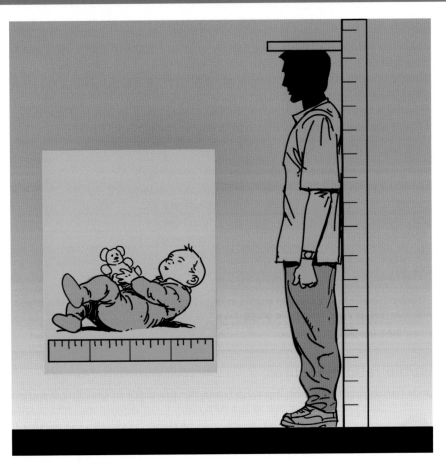

Figure 3.27 Measuring height

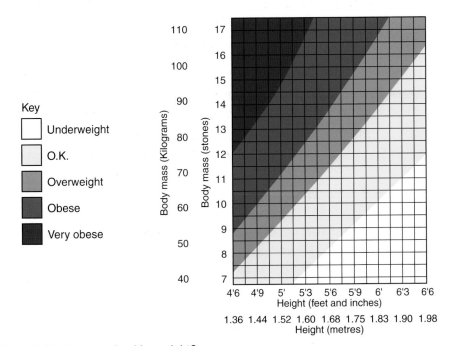

Figure 3.28 Are you a healthy weight?

This means that to calculate your BMI you should:

i) Use your calculator to find the square of your height in metres (for example, a height of 1.63 m will have a squared value of $1.63 \times 1.63 = 2.82$ m^2).

ii) Divide your mass in kg by the value calculated in step (i). This gives you your BMI.

iii) Compare your calculated BMI with the values given below in Table 3.9 (There are many websites that will do these calculations for you.)

Body mass index	Interpretation
Below 20	Underweight
20–25	Ideal weight
25–30	Overweight
30–40	Obese
Above 40	Grossly obese

Note: Research projects which would involve asking people their weights should be avoided, as some may feel very uncomfortable giving this information.

Table 3.9 BMI values

Waist/hip ratio measures

Research has shown that waist/hip ratio is a better predictor of deciding if someone is obese and at risk of having heart disease than the traditional BMI method. People can be either 'apple shaped' (with a lot of fat stored around their middles) or 'pear shaped' (with fat stored around their bottom and thighs). Apple-shaped people are more likely to develop heart disease than pear-shaped people. The waist/hip ratio shows whether you are an 'apple' or a 'pear'.

You can work out your waist-to-hip-ratio by dividing the measurement of your waist by that of your hips (there are many websites that will do this for you).

$$\text{i.e: waist/hip ratio} = \frac{\text{waist measurement}}{\text{hip measurement}}$$

For men, ideally the ratio should not be over 0.9.

For women, ideally the ratio should not be over 0.85.

The higher the ratio, the greater the risk of heart disease and strokes. If your ratio is over one, you are at significant risk.

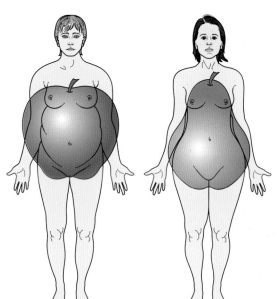

Figure 3.29 People can be either 'apple shaped' or 'pear shaped'

Body fat composition

The amount of body fat a person has can affect health).

Skin fold test

The simplest way of measuring body fat is using a skin fold test (see Figure 3.30). There is a layer of fat under the skin (subcutaneous fat). A caliper is used to pinch the skin at various points on the body and a gauge on the caliper measures the thickness of the pinch.

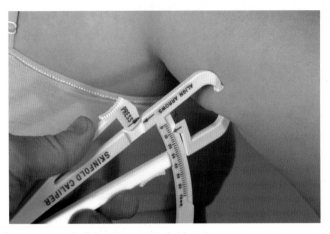

Figure 3.30 Measuring body fat using a skin fold test

ACTIVITY

If you can obtain calipers, have a go at doing a skin fold test.

● Take readings on the right side of the body.
● Pick up the skin fold between the thumb and forefinger, so that you are measuring two layers of skin and the subcutaneous fat. Place the calipers about one centimeter from the fingers and at a depth about equal to the thickness of the fold.
● Repeat this measurement three times (in mm) and calculate an average.
● The usual places on the body that are measured are shown in Figure 3.31
● Calculators can be found on the internet which will convert skin fold measurements to percentage body fat (for example, www.brianmac.co.uk/fatcent.htm)

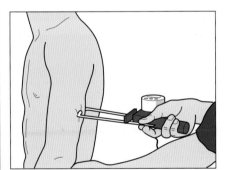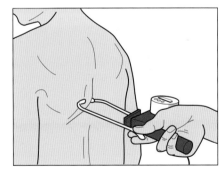

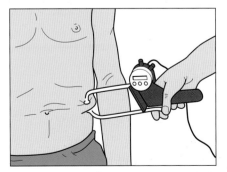

Figure 3.31 The sites shown may be used to determine body fat

Bioelectrical impedance

Most health professionals now use a method of measuring body fat called bioelectrical impedance. The person has sensors placed on their feet and/or hands. A very low level electrical signal is passed through the body, and the length of time it takes for the signal to pass between two sensors is recorded. Muscle tissue contains more water than fat, so it is a better conductor than body fat. This means the signal will travel quicker in a person with low body fat, and slower in a person with high body fat. The machine will give a read out of the body fat percentage.

Cholesterol level

What is cholesterol?

Cholesterol is a fat that occurs naturally in the body. People usually think of cholesterol as harmful. However, it has important uses in the body; for example, it is used for making:

- hormones, such as some sex hormones
- cell membranes
- bile salts (needed for digestion).

The cholesterol that we need is either obtained from our diet or made by the liver. Most cholesterol is transported as low density lipid proteins (LDLs). Too much LDL can cause the build up of cholesterol in the arteries, leading to coronary vascular diseases (CVD), such as a heart attack or stroke. Because of this, LDLs are sometimes known as 'bad cholesterol'.

Some cholesterol is transported as high density lipid proteins (HDLs). These can prevent the build up of cholesterol in the arteries, so HDLs are sometimes known as 'good cholesterol'.

A high level of total cholesterol (TC) is not good for health, and sometimes this is what is measured. However, often it is thought to be more useful to look at the relative amounts of HDL and LDL. It is healthier to have high HDL and low LDL. In other words, a low TC:HDL ratio is preferred when cholesterol levels are measured.

- The amount of total cholesterol in the blood can range from 3.6–7.8 mmol/l. (Units are millimoles per litre of blood).
- It is recommended that total cholesterol should be under 5 mmol/l, and LDL under 3 mmol/l.
- In the UK, two in three adults have a total cholesterol level of over 5 mmol/l.
- Women have, on average, a higher level of cholesterol than men (5.6 mmol/l compared with an average of 5.5 mmol/l in men).

Measuring cholesterol

Cholesterol can be measured with a simple blood test. Usually, the person would be asked not to eat for the 12 hours before, and then a small sample of blood will be taken, using a finger prick or a syringe. Home testing kits are available, but they may not be very accurate, plus there are many other factors that can increase the risk of heart disease, so it is important to talk about the results with a health professional.

Cholesterol tests are recommended for anyone who:

- has had any cardiovascular disease (CVD)
- has a family history of high blood cholesterol (hypercholesterolaemia)
- is over 35 and has one or more risk factor for coronary heart disease (i.e. family history of CVD, diabetes, high blood pressure, smokes).

> **KEY TERM**
>
> **Cardiovascular disease (CVD)** – disease of heart or circulation, for example atherosclerosis (narrowing of arteries), angina, coronary heart disease, stroke.

What can be done to lower the level of cholesterol?

- Eat a diet low in fats, particularly saturated fats; for example, cut down on animal fats such as red meat, butter and other dairy products and eggs.
- Eat five portions of fruit and vegetables a day which will provide plenty of fibre. Soluble fibre is thought to lower cholesterol level.
- Increase your level of exercise.
- Try to avoid being overweight.
- Foods can be bought (for example, some types of margarine) that contain ingredients to lower cholesterol, although these may be expensive.
- For certain people, for example those with signs of cardiovascular disease, health professionals may prescribe medicines, for example, statins.

Blood glucose tests

People who have type 1 diabetes need to regularly test their blood sugar (glucose) level. This will indicated whether they are managing their diabetes correctly. Maintaining a constant blood sugar level will both keep a person feeling well and reduce the chance of long term complications.

Blood glucose levels can be monitored by a person in their own home quickly and with very little discomfort. A finger-stick test using a blood glucose meter measures the level of sugar in the blood (see Figure 3.32).

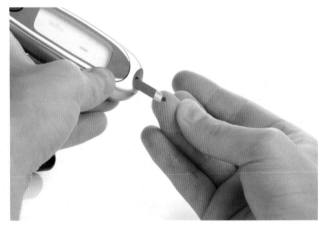

Figure 3.32 Testing blood sugar level

1. The finger is pricked with a small sharp needle (lancet).
2. A drop of blood is put on a test strip.
3. The test strip is put in a meter that displays the blood sugar level.

Meters can:

- provide readings within 15 seconds
- store the information for future use
- calculate an average blood glucose level over a period of time.

Some meters:

- display information as graphs or charts
- have spoken instructions and larger displays for the visually impaired
- can test sites other than the finger tips.

Liver function tests

The liver (Figure 3.33) is one of the largest organs in the body and carries out a wide range of functions.

Liver function tests (LFTs) measure chemicals in the blood that are made by the liver. If there is an abnormal level of any of these chemicals, it indicates that there may be a problem with liver function. A syringe with a fine needle is used to take a small volume of blood from a vein in the arm. The blood is sent to a laboratory to be tested. The laboratory will inform the health professional if the test forms within the normal range or not. 'Abnormal' results are not uncommon and will mean that further health tests will be carried out.

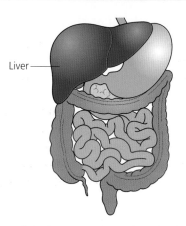

Figure 3.33 The liver is one of the largest organs of the body

Common liver function tests

- Total protein (all the proteins in the blood)
- Albumin (a type of protein)
- Liver enzymes
- Bilirubin (formed from the breakdown of haemoglobin from old red blood cells. A high level of bilirubin in the blood makes the skin appear yellowish – jaundiced)
- Clotting studies (tests to check that blood is clotting normally).

What the tests can show

Liver function tests often give one of the first indications of a disease of the liver.

- The tests can suggest what disease a person may have, for example hepatitis. They can also indicate liver damage or long-term alcohol abuse.
- The tests can show the severity of a disease.
- The tests can show if medication has side effects which affect liver function.

Resting pulse rate and recovery pulse rates after exercise

The pumping action of the heart causes a regular pulsation in the blood flow. This can be felt by pressing two finger tips against, either the wrist just below the base of the thumb (Figure 3.34) or, on the neck, a few centimetres below the jaw. It is often most convenient to count for 15 seconds and multiply by four to calculate the number of beats per minute. The pulse rate corresponds to the heart rate, which varies according to the person's state of relaxation or physical activity.

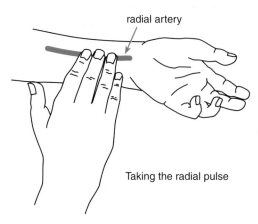

radial artery

Taking the radial pulse

Figure 3.34 How to locate the pulse at the wrist

Resting pulse rate

The resting pulse rate is the pulse rate taken after a period of relaxation. It should be taken at least three times and an average (mean) calculated. A low resting pulse rate generally indicates a better physical fitness level than a higher resting pulse rate.

- In reasonably fit individuals their pulse rate will be between 60 and 80 beats per minute, and on average 72 beats per minute in adults.
- In children and the elderly it will be higher than in young adults.
- Men, on average, have lower pulse rates than women.
- In top distance athletes it could be as low as 40 beats per minute.

Recovery after exercise

Another way of using pulse rate as an indicator of the level of a person's physical fitness is to see how quickly a person recovers and gets back to their own normal pulse rate after a period of exercise.

ACTIVITY

(**Important**: Don't attempt this activity if there are any reasons why you should not do moderate exercise.)

Equipment: step/bench/or box 50 cm high; stop watch

Work in pairs.

1. One person (A) takes the pulse of their partner (B), who should be relaxed, rested and sitting down. (See instructions above for taking resting pulse rate.)
2. Person B then does one minute of exercise. For example, they could step up and down on the step or walk quickly up and down stairs.
3. Person A takes their partner's pulse rate for 15 seconds immediately they have finished exercising, and records this as beats per minute (multiply by 4) in Table 3.10.
4. Person A continues to take their partner's pulse rate for 15 seconds every minute until the pulse rate returns to the resting rate.
5. The table will show recovery time, in other words, how many minutes it takes for the person's pulse rate to return to normal after exercise.
6. You could plot recovery rate on a graph. To do this you would plot pulse rate (y axis) against time (x axis) on a line graph. In a different colour you plot the resting rate as a horizontal straight line.
7. Compare the recovery rates of different volunteers. Can you explain the results you find? For example, does the person who recovers quickest do more exercise?

Resting pulse rate (i.e. before exercise):	
Time after exercise (minutes)	Pulse rate (beats per minute)
0 (i.e. straight after exercise)	
1	
2	
3 etc.	

Table 3.10

How to present conclusions from health and well-being assessments and make reasoned judgements

Making reasoned judgements

As you will have seen from the examples above, measurements of physical health must be compared with accepted normal values (or **norms**). These values will have been obtained by measuring many healthy people.

There is usually a **range** of values that is considered normal, not just one figure. In other words, health professionals will be checking if the subject's result falls between the highest and lowest healthy values. If it does not fall within this range, it would be considered abnormal.

It is important that other factors that may affect a value are taken into consideration when deciding whether a value is within normal limits or is abnormal; for example, the age of the person, or if they are male or female.

How to present conclusions from health and well-being assessments

When giving a person the results of a measurement of their physical health, they must be given a full explanation to show how they compare with normal values, and help and support if their values are considered abnormal.

This means that the following points will be important when presenting conclusions:

- **Adequate time** must be given, so that both a detailed explanation can be given and the subject has a **chance to ask questions**.
- Feedback must be given in an **appropriate place**; for example, it must be somewhere that the subject and person giving the conclusions will not be disturbed.
- The conclusions must be pitched at the **correct level**, using **appropriate language** to ensure that the subject understands the explanation.
- Sometimes it may be useful to show **images, such as graphs or tables** to show how the results compare with normal values.
- There may be **issues of confidentiality**. When using a person as the subject of a case study, it is often best to use a different name. Before taking any measurements, it must be made clear to the subject who will have access to the results.
- When giving results that are either higher or lower than normal values, it is important to **motivate** people to change, **not to stress or frighten** them.
- If results are significantly different from normal values and the apparatus and methods used are reliable, it may be advisable to suggest that the person sees a health professional for the measurement to be checked.

How results of assessments will be used to develop realistic health improvement plans for an individual or a group of individuals

The section below, '*Promoting and supporting health improvement*', guides you through using the results of health assessments to design health and well-being improvement plans for individuals, or groups of individuals.

Promoting and supporting health improvement

Designing a health and well-being improvement plan for an individual or group of individuals

Stages in the development of a health improvement plan

1. The health status of a person, or group, must be assessed. This may be from:

    -   physical measures of health
        Measurements of blood pressure; peak flow; body mass index; waist to hip ratios; body fat composition; cholesterol levels and pulse rate at rest and after exercise may all be useful indicators of physical health status. (see *'Indicators of physical health'* on pages 170–179, above).
    -   lifestyle information
        This will be used to make an assessment of all aspects of health – physical, intellectual, social and emotional.

    As much information as possible must be gathered on lifestyle and indicators of physical health (measurements) to allow the health risks of an individual or a group to be identified.

2. Resources must be identified.
    What health promotion materials are available to inform, motivate and support people to improve their health and well-being? For example, which organisations, books, leaflets, posters, advertisements and websites will provide useful health promotion materials? Useful materials can be obtained from GPs, NHS, Health Education Centres, Health Promotion Units, and local organisations.

    This is important as a health plan will only work if the individual is motivated. They must want to change (Figure 3.35).

3. The health and well-being improvement plan is designed.
    The plan should consider physical, intellectual, emotional and social health. Methods and activities must be planned to bring about the necessary improvements identified. How will the individual have to change their behaviour to bring about the health improvement targets?

    The person putting the plan together needs empathy for the feelings of the person for whom the plan has been created, and understands that a person's choice about their health and well-being can be affected by self-esteem, financial factors and social pressures. The plan should be appropriate to the individual; for example, it would be useless to suggest membership of an expensive gym to a person who was not well-off, or very vigorous exercise to an elderly person.

    The plan, including the language used, should reflect the needs and abilities of the chosen subject, for example, child, adolescent, adult or elderly person.

4. Realistic short- and long-term targets must be set.
    What health improvements are aimed for and in what time scale? The plan should include short-term and long-term targets with time scales. For example, a short-term target could be to increase physical activity, such as walking to work three times a week. In the long-term this would improve levels of fitness and weight loss, so a long-term target could be to lower resting pulse rate to 75 beats per minute, or a weight loss of 4 kg.

    Targets should be realistic. For example, a very rapid weight loss is likely to be unrealistic. An exercise programme should start gently, and then gradually build up.

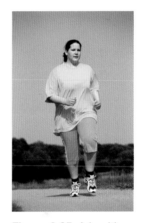

Figure 3.35 A health plan will only work if the individual wants to change

5. **An assessment of the difficulties that may be experienced in implementing (carrying out) the health and well-being improvement plan must be made.**

   The weaknesses of the plan should be identified. It is important to remember that activities to improve health, such as dieting and increasing exercise, involve determination from the person following the plan. It is likely that some parts of the plan will be more challenging to achieve than other parts and these should be anticipated with practical suggestions made of how to overcome difficulties.

6. **An assessment of the support available in the implementation of the health and well-being improvement plan must be made.**

   It can be very difficult for individuals to maintain their motivation. At the start they may be enthusiastic and change their behaviour, but they may find this hard to sustain, particularly if they do not see immediate improvements in their health.

   - It will be very helpful to them to have friends or family who can give encouragement when they are struggling.
   - In some cases, it will be helpful for family or friends to join them, for example, in their exercise routine or giving up smoking.
   - It may be that the individual may be dependent on others to a certain extent, and so will need their cooperation in making changes. A teenager, for example, is likely to eat at least some of their meals with the rest of the family, so the cooperation of those who shop and cook would help them make their diet healthier.

To produce the health plan for an individual

Introduction

- Identify the individual who is to be the focus of the health plan. It must be someone who wants to maintain or improve their health and well-being. Check that they are happy for you to share their personal information with other people, providing you maintain confidentiality by using a different name.
- Measure relevant indicators of physical health, for example, blood pressure; peak flow; body mass index; waist to hip ratios; body fat composition; cholesterol levels and pulse rate at rest and after exercise.
- Do relevant calculations, for example, BMI (page 171); waist-to-hip ratios (page 174) and resting pulse rate (page 179).
- Explain the differences between the individual's state of health and recommended norms.
- Identify any lifestyle factors that are having a positive effect on physical, intellectual, emotional and social health.
- Explain how these factors interrelate to positively affect the individual's health.
- Identify risks to physical, intellectual, emotional and social health, highlighting those over which the individual may have control.
- Find which aspect of their physical, intellectual, emotional and social health they are most concerned about.
- Analyse your findings, taking into consideration the individual's age, sex and lifestyle.

The Health Plan

- Identify the improvements that you will focus on.
- Prioritise long- and short-term targets for improvement, including timescales.

- Explain the impact on their health should the person achieve the targets.
- Explain possible risks to the individual if targets are not achieved and how they could damage health in both the short and long term.
- Explain in a way appropriate to your chosen person, how they can change their behaviour to meet the targets.

In conclusion
- Explain why the health plan is relevant for this individual.
- Identify potential difficulties in following and achieving the plan.
- Explain the support that might be required and is available for the individual to achieve their goals.
- Select health promotional materials, and keep a bibliography.

To produce the health plan for a group of individuals

A health plan can be aimed at a group of individuals. The steps described above can be adapted to improve the health of a number of people with a common lifestyle and common health problems. Working together to improve health may give people increased motivation, as demonstrated by many weight loss clubs (see Figure 3.36).

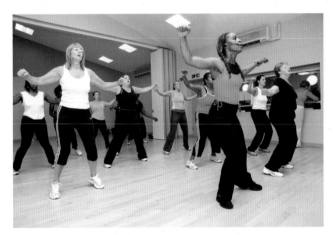

Figure 3.36 Working towards improved health as a group, can increase the motivation of individuals

GLOSSARY

Amniocentesis – a test in which some of the amniotic fluid that surrounds the baby in the womb is removed to test for genetic disorders
Asthma – disease in which there is narrowing of the airways, leading to wheezing, coughing, tightness of the chest and shortness of breath
Blood glucose test – measurement of glucose level in blood
Blood pressure – the pressure at which blood flows through the circulatory system
Body mass index (BMI) – a simple assessment of body mass.

$$BMI = \frac{body\ mass/kg}{(height/m)^2}$$

GLOSSARY – (continued)

Bronchitis – disease in which the small airways are blocked and damaged, leading to a severe cough producing large quantities of phlegm (a mix of mucus, bacteria and white blood cells)

Carcinogen – cancer causing chemical (e.g. in tar found in cigarettes)

Cardiovascular diseases – conditions that affect the heart and circulation

Cholesterol – a fat that occurs naturally in the body; can build up in arteries, causing heart disease

Chorionic villus sampling (CVS) – a test in which some of the placenta is removed to test for genetic disorders in the baby

Culture – shared values based on beliefs, practice, dress, language, diet and religion

Disease – a specific condition of ill health, identified as an actual change on the surface or inside some part of the body (Compare with **Illness**)

DNA (deoxyribonucleic acid) – the molecule that forms the genetic material

Emotional health – concerned with the ability to recognise emotions such as fear, joy, grief, frustration and anger, and to express such emotions appropriately

Emphysema – disease in which there is breakdown of air sacs in the lungs, leading to wheezing and shortness of breath.

Ethnicity – a shared identity that comes from a common culture, religion or tradition

Gender – the psychological and social development of male and female roles in a society

Holistic – looking at the whole system rather than just concentrating on individual components

Illness – the subjective state of feeling unwell (i.e. how people feel) (Compare with Disease)

Intellectual health – concerned with the ability to think clearly and rationally

Liver function test (LFT) – measure of chemicals in blood made by liver

Mutation – an unpredictable change in genetic material.

Nicotine – drug in tobacco that causes addiction and increases heart rate and blood pressure

Obesity – the excessive deposit of fat under the skin.

Objective – based on facts, not personal feelings or opinions

Peak flow – a measure of how fast you can blow air out of your lungs.

Physical health – concerned with the physical functioning of the body

Poverty – lack of resources helping you to be healthy

Pulse – regular pulsation in blood flow through arteries

Recovery pulse rate – time taken for pulse to return to normal rate after exercise

Relative poverty – a lack of resources (income) sufficient to achieve a standard of living considered acceptable in a society

Respiratory diseases – conditions that affect breathing, such as asthma and bronchitis

GLOSSARY – (continued)

Rural area – a sparsely populated area; as well as agricultural areas, rural areas include 'honey pot' villages that rely heavily on tourism, urban fringe commuter villages and former coal-mining communities

Screening – a simple test carried out on a large number of apparently healthy people to separate those who probably have a certain disease from those who do not.

Social exclusion – when an individual is prevented from taking part in any of the key economic, social and political activities in the society in which they live

Social health – concerned with the ability to relate to others and to form relationships with other people

Socio-economic group – category people are put in depending on their social class, wealth and income and education

Sphygmomanometer – equipment used for measuring blood pressure

Stress – the inability to cope with change

Subjective – based on an individual's point of view

Urban area – town or city

Vaccine – a preparation given to a person to stimulate their white blood cells to produce antibodies, so that they will not develop a disease when they come in contact with the bacteria or virus that causes it.

Waist/hip ratio

$$= \frac{\text{Waist measurement}}{\text{Hip measurement}}$$

CHAPTER 4

Health, Social Care and Early Years in Practice

CHAPTER CONTENT

This chapter will help you learn about:
- the range of care needs of major client groups
- the care values commonly used in practitioner work
- the development of self-concept and personal relationships
- promoting and supporting health improvement

Care workers in health, social care and early years services need a comprehensive knowledge and understanding of the core principles that underpin their work. This chapter will develop your knowledge and understanding of some of the core principles that were explained in the first three chapters.

This unit is externally assessed and will cover the settings in which care takes place and the service users who access the services in these settings. You would find it useful to keep a file of items relating to this chapter that could help you in the assessment.

The range of care needs of the major client groups

Throughout this book we have focused on the client groups shown in Table 4.1 and Figure 4.1.

We have also identified the needs of service users and the range of care needs of the major client groups (see Table 4.2).

Life Stage	Age Span
Infancy	0–2 years
Early childhood	3–8 years
Adolescence	9–18 years
Early adulthood	19–45 years
Middle adulthood	46–65
Later adulthood	66+

Table 4.1 Six main life stages

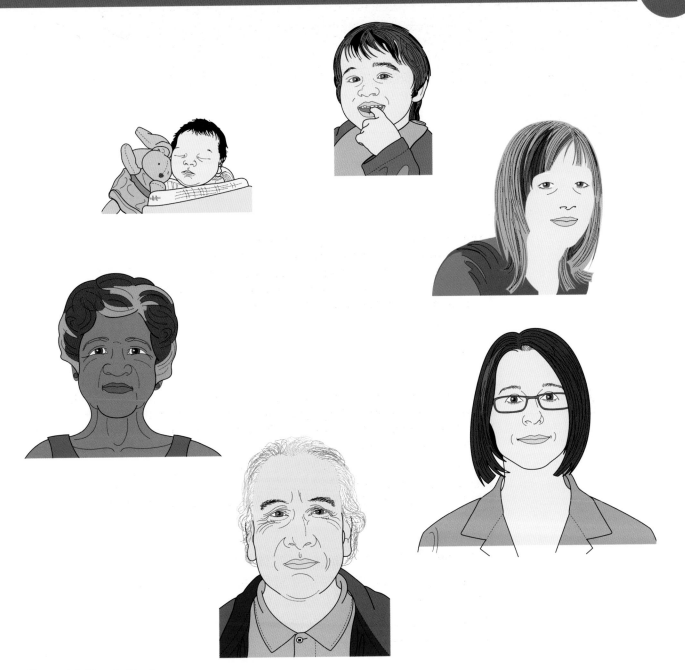

Figure 4.1 The six life stages

Physical needs	Basic needs of humans such as food, water, shelter and clothing
Intellectual needs	The ability to learn and to develop new skills
Emotional needs	The expression of feelings, giving and receiving love and security
Social needs	The ability to develop and maintain relationships, including friendships, intimate and sexual relationships, and work relationships

Table 4.2 The basic needs of service users split into the following areas

ACTIVITY

Look at the following case studies and decide which basic needs are not being met and suggest ways practitioners could help these clients meet their needs. Building on the work you did in Chapter 2, think of which health and care practitioners could help.

CASE STUDIES

Case Study 1

Eric sleeps rough on the streets. He came out of the army and became homeless. One night he was beaten up and ended up in the local A & E. His wounds were cleaned up. The staff had a discussion about what they should do for him.

Case Study 2

Nancy is 5. Her family are travellers and they have recently moved to a new site in Surrey. Because the family have always been on the move, Nancy has never gone to school.

Case Study 3

Bernadette has learning disabilities. She is 19 and is about to leave college where she has been on a catering course (NVQ level 1). Her social worker has found her a flat where she will live with three other women with learning disabilities. She is nervous about leaving her parents and living away from them, although she wants to become more independent. At the moment she stays in her room most of the time and looks at the TV. She has tried to make friends at the college, but she is very shy.

Case Study 4

Harold is 80. His wife, Maggie, died last year. They had been together for over 50 years and he misses her a lot. His family want him to move into sheltered housing, where he will have company and help with cooking and household chores.

Case Study 5

Alice (15) has had a baby, George, who is now 3-months-old. Alice lives with her mother (Eileen) in a flat on a social housing estate in South London. Alice finds it difficult to cope with the baby; she bottle feeds him and often he vomits after his bottle. George seems to cry a lot and he is not putting on any weight.

We can see from these examples that we all have basic needs throughout our lives. Eric needs shelter, but he also needs friendships and to feel part of the society he lives in.

When we think about the basic needs of these five people and who may help, we also need to be aware that professionals dealing with their clients have to be aware that clients have rights and may not agree with the professionals' view about 'what is best for them'.

Harold may prefer to stay in the house he has lived in for years, with the neighbours and friends he has, than move to a new flat, where he is in a different area and away from the house with all its memories.

Eric may be quite annoyed that the staff – who don't know him – are deciding what 'to do' with him, without asking him what he wants to do.

At the same time, children's services focus on the needs of the child, and if Alice is unable to care for George, the services will try to support Alice so that she becomes more confident in looking after her baby. If this is not possible, George may be taken into care so that George's needs are met, either by placing him with a foster carer or possibly adoption.

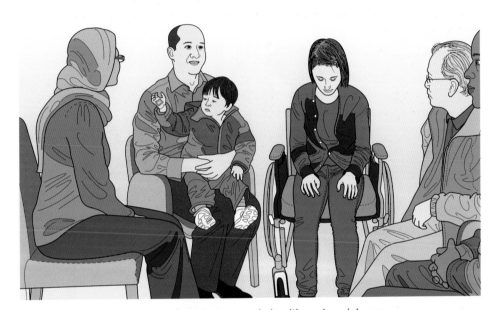

Figure 4.2 There are a range of services users in health and social care

Now we are going to look at some of the needs people have in more detail.

Physical needs

The basic needs of human beings such as food, water, shelter and clothing.

Food

A recent campaign called 'Hungry to be Heard' by Age Concern highlighted the problem of malnourishment in hospitals. The organisation found that six out of ten people are at risk of becoming malnourished in hospital. All patients who receive good nutrition when they are in hospital may have shorter hospital stays, fewer post-operative complications, and less need for drugs and other treatments. Age Concern outlined the following seven steps to end malnutrition in hospitals:

1. Hospital staff must listen to patients, their relatives and carers and act on what they say (this could be about food choice related to religion, or ability to chew or swallow).
2. All ward staff must become food aware (this could be about staff knowing which foods are most nutritious and easily digested for patients).

3. Hospital staff must follow their own professional codes and guidance from other bodies.
4. Older people must be assessed for the signs or danger of malnourishment on admission and at regular intervals during their stay.
5. Protected meal times should be introduced (this means that hospital staff, including, doctors should not be in the ward, talking to patients or assessing them during meal time).
6. Hospitals should introduce a red tray system. This means that vulnerable patients who need help with feeding should have their meal placed on a red tray so staff are aware that this person needs help with feeding.
7. Volunteers could be used to assist with feeding.

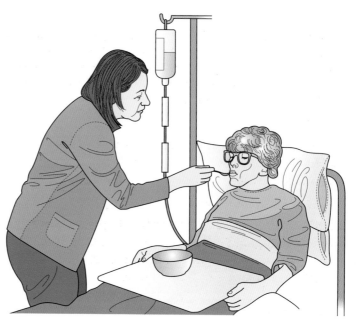

Figure 4.3 It is important that in-patients have enough to eat

These are some of the findings of the Age Concern study 'Hungry to be Heard':

1. A 79-year-old man was admitted to hospital, following a fall. He was given no help or encouragement to eat. He had Parkinson's Disease (a neurological disease which affects a person's mobility and there is often shaking and tremor in the limbs, which makes it difficult to eat or lift a cup of tea). After discussions with his family, he was given pureed food and fortified drinks, but when he left hospital he had lost a lot of weight.
2. A Mr P was admitted to hospital for an urgent heart operation. He suffered from coeliac disease and was unable to digest gluten. The hospital provided various meals for special diets but not for coeliac disease. He was also allergic to onions and eggs, which would give him severe pain.
3. Mrs J (83) was admitted to hospital after an accident at home. She had lost weight before her admission and her family were worried about her. The hospital had a sign saying 'If you feel that your relative needs assistance during mealtimes you are welcome to come in and assist us'.

DISCUSSION

What do you think of these stories? Several groups that need care could be at risk of malnourishment or malnutrition. People with learning disabilities or mental illness, infants and small children have to have their food and fluid intake monitored carefully. If older people have limited fluids, they are more at risk from urinary infections and other problems. What do you think of the hospital putting up a notice asking relatives to feed their family members? Whose responsibility is it to ensure people in health and social care settings have enough to eat and drink?

These issues relate to the principles of care that all practitioners should follow.

KEY TERM

Malnutrition – a disorder brought about by an inadequate diet or lack of food which causes physical deterioration. Malnourishment is sometimes used to mean the same.

Some hospitals now use the MUST tool to monitor patients who may be at risk for malnourishment. MUST stands for the Malnutrition Universal Screening Tool. This means patients are regularly weighed during their stay in the hospital ward and their food and fluid intake is monitored. There are NICE guidelines that state how the nutrition of patients should be carried out

The NICE guidelines state:

- Nutritional screening should be carried out by trained staff.
- Nutritional support should be given to people who are malnourished.
- Swallowing problems should be identified.

The NICE guidelines also state that:

- All health care professionals directly involved in patient care should receive education and training on the importance of providing adequate nutrition.
- Nutritional support should be carried out by the multi-disciplinary team.
- Acute hospitals should have a nutrition nurse.

KEY TERM

NICE – the National Institute for Excellence. NICE recommends what drugs should be used in the NHS and also what treatments for a range of conditions are effective.

Diet and sick children

Children who are ill often have poor appetites. A few days without food will not harm the chid as long as the fluid intake is increased.

- Encourage the child to drink a range of fluids – fruit juice, water, milk or soups.
- Bendy straws or feeding beakers may be used.
- Drinks should be offered at frequent intervals to prevent dehydration.
- Try to make the food as attractive as possible.
- Do not overload the plate – you can always give a second helping.
- Give foods that are easy to manage, yoghurts etc, that do not need chewing.

Some children may be on special diets. You would be given details of this and it is important you follow the instructions.

There has been an increase in diabetes among children under 16.

Children with cystic fibrosis need a diet high in fats.

Children with coeliac disease need a gluten-free diet.

Children who have problems swallowing need a soft or liquid diet.

As we have mentioned before, more children are obese, so these children will have a diet that is low in fat and sugar and high in high fibre carbohydrates.

We can see from this section that adequate and appropriate intake of food and drink is a key issue for health and care practitioners and for those working with babies and young children.

Intellectual needs

In Chapters 1 and 2 we saw how the development of intellectual skills is important for our personal development throughout our lives. In Chapter 2 we saw that children in care do less well at school and this affects their choice of job, housing and general welfare. The Department for Children, Schools and Families is responsible for children in care and they have outlined 'Time to Deliver', a practical guide for local authorities to improve the chances of these children. Looked after children are less likely to go to university and more likely to end up in prison. The Children and Young People legislation will make it a legal requirement for:

- schools to have a designated teacher to help children in care reach their full potential
- social workers will visit all looked after children and support them
- local authorities to give children in care financial support if they go on to higher education
- local authorities will appoint personal advisers to help older children.

Intellectual needs are not just about doing well at school and going on to university. Many groups that are supported by workers in health and social care may be limited in their abilities because of disability or illness. However, this does not mean their intellectual needs should be ignored.

Look at the following examples:

EXAMPLE

- Katy is 19 and has a mental age of 7. She has learning disabilities and attends the local FE college, where she is taking an NVQ course in child care.
- Peter is 50. He had a bad car accident and is paralysed from the neck down. He uses a voice recognition computer and he paints using a brush held in his mouth.

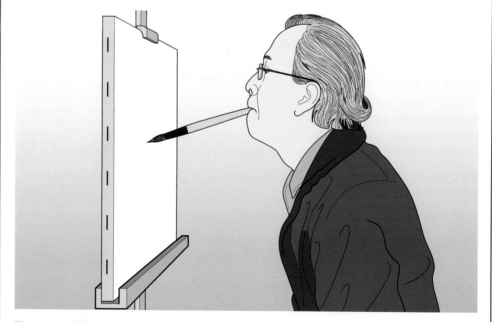

Figure 4.4 Whatever happens to us we still have intellectual needs

(continued)

EXAMPLE – (continued)

- Edwina is 45. She was born with CP (Cerebral Palsy). Her speech is difficult to understand. She uses a wheelchair. She has enrolled on an Open University course.

Using our intellectual abilities helps us in our personal development and also gives us a sense of self-worth. When care workers are assessing people in residential care they usually ask about their hobbies and interests. In some homes there may be a scrabble or puzzle club.

Emotional needs

We all need to feel loved or cared for, but this may be a problem for certain groups.

EXAMPLES

Example 1
Karen (30) lives in a hostel for young people with learning disabilities. She is very fond of a boy she met at a day centre. She asked the manager of the home if Peter could go up to her room. The manager is worried about what may happen if Karen has a sexual relationship, as she is very vulnerable and immature.

Example 2
Myra's husband died many years ago and she still really misses male company. She goes to a lunch club one day a week. They have tea dances some weeks. The women dress up and there is ballroom dancing. Myra is 75 and feels she is too old for 'all that stuff', but she enjoys the physical contact in dancing.

Example 3
Sam is 14. He has Obsessive Compulsive Disorder (OCD) which means he is always washing his hands and rearranging the things in his work bag, which means he is often late for school. Sam's mother is divorced and she has a lot of boyfriends. She never seems to have time for Sam.

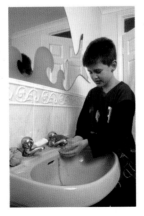

Figure 4.5 OCD can affect your daily life

(continued)

EXAMPLES – (continued)

Example 4

Tim (40) trained as a carer for people with learning disabilities. He enjoyed the work but he wanted a job with more variety. He trained as a masseur. Sometimes he gives hand massages to older people in residential homes. The older residents tell him that no one ever touches them or hugs them any more and they really miss the contact. They find that the hand massages Tim does make them feel much better and relaxed.

If you work in health and social care, it is important to think about how we use touch. Is it just to guide someone down the corridor? Many carers use touch to reassure patients; for example, they may hold their hand when they have an examination. Who touches you and how does that make you feel? We also need to be aware that in some cultures, touching is seen as a very intimate action and should only be done by a spouse or close family member. Some sheltered housing schemes allow residents to bring their pet with them. Research has shown that having a cat or dog and showing it affection can improve your health and reduce your blood pressure. It also helps if the pet shows affection back to the owner!

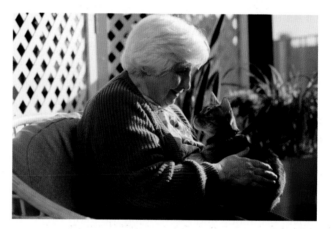

Figure 4.6 Pets are good for your health!

Social needs

Relationships and friendships are very important for our emotional well-being. We have seen examples of this in Chapter 1. Relationships occur throughout our lives. Research has shown that people with 10 or more friends are happier than those with 5 or less.

Work relationships are important when you are a health or social care practitioner. The ability to work as part of a team is vital in departments such as the operating theatre, the maternity ward and in Accident & Emergency. The care of our patients and clients is dependent on our ability to work with colleagues. In Chapter 2 we saw that the efficient working of a multi-disciplinary team can make a difference to patient care.

Many clients we have in health and social care may have social needs that cannot be met because, either their relatives have died, or live far away. In residential homes every effort is made for residents to keep in touch with friends and family, via the phone in the home or by visits. There may be outings to the pub or shopping centre arranged. Local churches and voluntary organisations can also play a part in providing social support to clients.

EXAMPLE 1

An advocacy service was set up by a voluntary group in a London borough. The purpose of the group was to help people deal with issues in their lives, such as the death of a partner, money worries, or problems with neighbours. Initially, it was decided that the contact made with each client would be for six weeks. However, the volunteers found that the people they were helping were very lonely. They saw very few people. They often had mobility problems. Now the service has become a befriending service when a volunteer is matched with a client and regular visits and phone calls are made. In the evaluation of the service, all the clients said it made a big difference to their lives.

KEY TERM

Advocacy – an advocate supports a service user so that they can express their view and have a say in their care planning.

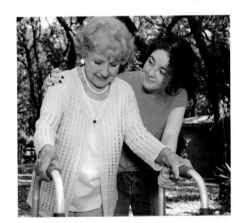

Figure 4.7 Everyone has social needs

There are examples of voluntary groups that offer social support to different groups. PHAB is one of these. This club offers social meetings for young people with and without disabilities.

We all have social needs and it is important that these are met.

In Chapter 1 we looked at examples of factors that affect human growth and development. We will look at some of these in more detail.

Life course events

Life course is a term used to describe events which happen to us during our lives. These events may be experienced by a large number of people – such as the Second World War or they could be events that only happen to a few people – illness, disability, unemployment or redundancy. As we have seen in Unit 1, most of us experience a range of life course events such as being in a family group, going to play group or nursery school, going to school, training or going to college, starting work, making relationships, getting married or divorced, and becoming old or experiencing ill-health. All these events have an impact on our personal development.

Holmes and Rahe (1967) developed a Social Readjustment Rating Scale which allocates a number of Life Crisis Units to different events. If you have a high score over two years, you may be at risk from mental or physical ill-health. If you have more than 300 LCUs in this time, you have an 80% chance of illness. Table 4.3 shows the LCUs s given to the top 10 events outlined by Holmes and Rahe.

Rank	Life event	Score
1	Death of spouse	100
2	Divorce	73
3	Marital separation	65
4	Jail term	63
5	Death of close family member	63
6	Personal injury or illness	53
7	Marriage	50
8	Fired at work	47
9	Marital reconciliation	45
10	Retirement	45

Table 4.3 The LCUs given to the top 10 events

This table just shows the top 10 of life events which may cause us stress. Can you think of things that have happened to you that have been stressful. Stressful events can be happy events – a new baby in the family – as well as sad events.

The full version of the table includes 43 events that have an effect on a person's development. These events included change in schools, Christmas, moving house and trouble with in laws! You could find the full table on the Internet.

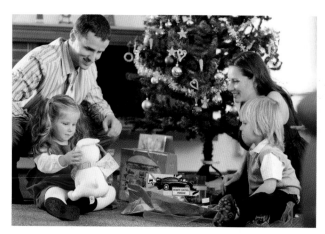

Figure 4.8 Even happy events can be stressful

Life events, such as those listed by Holmes and Rahe, are now more likely to be seen as processes we go through. Life events can cause initial reaction of shock or surprise, but they can also be used positively so that the event becomes part of our life and the way we see things, rather than dominating every second of out waking life. We saw in Chapter 1 (page 57) how the experience of a cot death can add to that parent's life so that the experience can be used in a positive way. A married woman who loses her husband becomes a 'widow' and a person who is disabled as a result of an accident is seen as 'a person with a disability'. Care workers need to be aware of the problem of giving labels to people they support. In the 1950s when a ward round was done, the consultant would refer to the patients not by name but by their condition. So Mrs Jones, became the appendix in Bed 2. When we are looking after people with certain illnesses, whether it is in their own home, in hospital or clinic, or in a care home, we must always be aware of the whole person and have a 'holistic' approach.

KEY TERM

Holistic approach – an approach that looks at the whole person, not just the disease or injury or diagnosis.

Lifestyle choices

As we have seen in Chapters 1 and 3, lifestyle choices are determined by many factors including: age, gender, social class, level of income, ethnicity, the area you live in, and your level of fitness.

Lifestyle choices could include things like:

- what you eat and drink
- where you go out at weekends
- what exercise you have – do you ride a bike, drive a car, play games of some kind?
- do you save money or do you spend it all?
- where you go on holiday
- what you do in your spare time.

Your choices can be limited by your age, the films you see and clubs you go to.

Your choices may be limited by the money you have and the amount of free time you have.

Do you have any real choice? Some people may feel they have limited choice of life style if they live in a boarding school, or residential home.

ACTIVITY

Make a list of all the things you do that you would say make up your life style. Discuss your list with the rest of your group. What things are the same and what things are different. Think about your parents' life style. How far is it the same as yours, and how far is it different?

Choice for service users

It is very important that service users of health and social care services are offered choice. This may be about the clothes they wear, the food they eat, or the activities they do. You can only make an informed choice if the options are really explained to you so that you can make a choice yourself, rather than do what the doctor or nurse tells you.

EXAMPLES

Example 1

If you have an operation the doctor must explain to you what the operation involves and what complications may occur. This should be done before you sign the consent form.

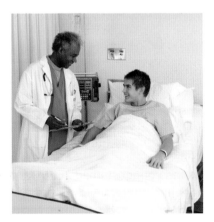

Figure 4.9 It is important that doctors give clear explanations to their patients so that they can make an informed choice

Example 2

You are 14 years old and you find out you are pregnant. You need to discuss all the options fully before making a decision what to do.

Example 3

Alma is 60 and she has been told she has cancer. She asks the doctor what treatment there is. He tells her that she can have chemotherapy, but he also tells her about the side effects of the drugs.

How expected and unexpected events impact on individuals during their life course

In Chapter 1 we have seen how expected and unexpected events impact on individuals. As health, social care and early years workers, we have to support service users through these changes.

Expected events

Starting school

This is a big event for the child and also the parent. Early years workers need to support both the child and the parent during this time.

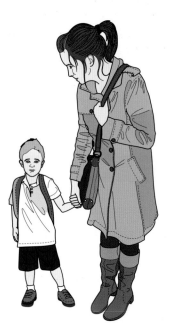

Figure 4.10 Sam starting school

CASE STUDY 2

Sam was 4 in July. He is the youngest child in the family; he had three brothers. According to the education policy in the area in which he lives, he starts full time school in September. His mother, Nicky, is worried because she feels he is too young to have a full day at school. He is a sensitive boy who would cry for his mother if she left him with babysitters. He has been in and out of hospital with asthma since he was a baby.

How could you make the experience of starting school less worrying for both Sam and his mother?

Marriage

Although marriage is about a couple making a commitment to each other, marriage also involves other members of both families.

CASE STUDY 3

Maria is 38 and she had almost given up hope of getting married. Her mother Liz kept on about her being an 'old maid'. Liz also kept on saying she wanted to be a granny. Maria met Paul at a local club. He had been married before and had a son Ross, who was 9 years old. Maria got on well with Ross, as they were both interested in football. Maria and Paul got engaged and decided to get married. The two sets of in-laws met. Maria felt that Paul's parents did not really approve of her. Paul's parents and Maria's parents did not get on. Liz said they were stuck-up. There were endless arguments about everything to do with the wedding. Paul and his parents drew up a list of guests and Liz disapproved of it. Paul and Maria wanted to have a quiet wedding with just a few friends but Liz wanted a big do, as her only daughter was getting married. Paul's ex-wife did not want Ross to be a page at the wedding. It became very difficult and Maria was always upset.

ACTIVITY

What advice would you give to:

● Maria and Paul
● Liz
● Paul's ex wife.

It is not surprising that marriage is put at number 7 on the social readjustment scale!

Partnership formation

Nowadays many people do not marry but cohabit instead – see Chapter 1 page 48.

Partnerships can be between single people, as well as between people who have had previous partnerships, with children from these previous relationships.

There are always problems with new partnerships between people who have ex-partners (see Chapter 1). The children can feel excluded now mum or dad are in a new relationship. Ex-wives and husbands can disapprove.

One new aspect of partnerships are civil partnerships.

Same-sex couples

Many same-sex couples live in stable relationships in the UK. Prejudice against same-sex couples has declined with the more liberal attitudes of people towards gay and lesbian people. This has developed further with the 'coming out' of well-known figures in entertainment and politics.

In December 2005 the Civil Partnership Act came into force in the UK. This allows civil marriages between same-sex couples to take place in register offices. The Civil Partnership allows same-sex couples to make a formal, legal commitment to each other by forming a civil partnership. Before the Act, same sex couples had a range of problems that heterosexual partners did not experience, especially those linked to inheritance when one partner dies.

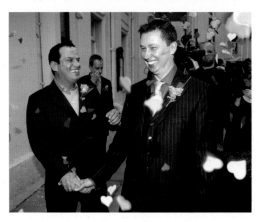

Figure 4.11 Civil partnerships are now legal in the UK

Same-sex couples may still experience homophobia and prejudice, but they are now able to take part in life events that were denied to them before.

Employment

Employment is a life event that most people expect to experience. However, employment is dependent on the economy of a society and the number of jobs that are available. In the 1950s many jobs were in the manufacturing industries: car manufacturing, making textiles in the mills and other production industries. Since the 1980s manufacturing has declined and most people are employed in the service sector. That is in shops, banks, building societies and health and social care. With the economic problems in 2008 we can no longer expect to be employed in the same job for a long time. Choice of where we work and what we do may be limited in the future and this will affect us emotionally and socially.

Death and bereavement

We all know we will die one day and we expect our grandparents and parents to die before us. We may be able to cope with death and bereavement better if we have a religion which can provide comfort. Sudden death of friends or family members can be difficult to cope with, especially if people die young. Death of a partner, close friend or family members scores highly on the Holmes and Rahe scale. How far we can cope with these events will be determined by the resources available to us. These may be social, such as the presence of family and friends in our social network; or they may be personal, such as our health, self-esteem and ability to cope. Sometimes it may be necessary to use professional help, such as a counselling or bereavement service.

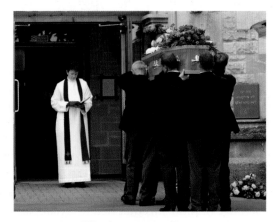

Figure 4.12 Bereavement can be difficult to cope with

During our lifetime we may also have to cope with unexpected events

Serious illness

A serious illness can have a long-term effect on our development.

CASE STUDY 5

Susanna and Rosie are sisters who are aged 18 and 16. They both have ME and they spend a lot of time in bed. Susanna had to reduce her attendance at school, as she was so weak and ill. She finally managed to get 2 GCSEs. Susanna always takes a long time to recover from the effort of going out. Last Christmas she went out to a restaurant with her friends, but then she was so exhausted she had to spend more and more time in bed. Her mother has to drive her everywhere. She uses a wheelchair as she is too weak to walk far. When Rosie became ill, her mother could not believe that both girls had the same problem. The GP has been very supportive, but he says he does not know much about ME. It is difficult to diagnose and treat, although research has been done in the USA to try to find out more about the disease. Rosie sometimes manages to spend a few hours a week in school.

KEY TERM

Myalgic encephalomyelitis (M.E) – sometimes called chronic fatigue syndrome (CFS) – is a disease when people have extreme fatigue, pains in their joints, and feel unwell.

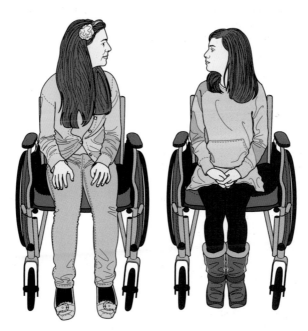

Figure 4.13 Illness can seriously affect your life

DISCUSSION

How do you think Susanna and Rosie have been affected by their illness? How has it affected their physical, intellectual, emotional and social development? They have been unable to take part in all the activities teenage girls should expect to do. They are unable to develop friends of either sex. They are still very dependent on their mother to help them. How do you think they feel about the future?

Relationship breakdown

We tend to think about relationship breakdown in couple relationships, including divorce, but there are many other types of relationship breakdowns. These could include the breakdown of the relationship between brothers or sisters; between mothers and sons or daughters; between different generations of the same family.

Financial difficulty

Sometimes financial difficulties can occur because people get into debt they cannot afford to repay, or because they are bad at managing money and spend it

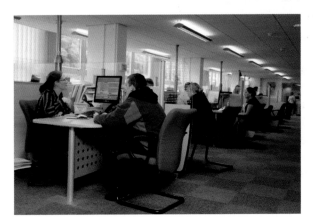

Figure 4.14 Being unemployed can affect your health and well-being

as soon as they get it. Sometimes people have financial difficulties because of factors that are beyond their control, like the Credit Crunch of 2008 when banks lent a lot of money to people who could not afford to repay it; this meant the banks were under pressure and everyone in society had difficulties as a result. If your problems are because it is your fault – you gambled the money away on the dogs or horses, you may learn from your mistakes and be more careful in the future. If the problems are caused by factors outside your control, you may feel very let down by society and the government. If you blame other people for your problems – even if that is the case – it is difficult to move on. Many people have been affected by the financial downturn of 2008. These are people who have saved carefully for the future; who bought a house they now find is worth less than they paid for it; who expected to send their children to private schools and have nice holidays. It is very difficult for people to accept this and their self-esteem and feelings of self-worth will be badly affected.

Loss of job

In recent years in the UK, most people who wanted employment were able to find it. Redundancy can have a bad effect on your self-esteem as we saw in Chapter 1 pages 55–6. Because of the 2008 economic downturn, many people in the City (London), who had earned high salaries and enjoyed large bonuses, were made redundant with little notice. These city banking workers earned a lot of money; had children at private schools; had expensive holidays and lived in large houses. Their wives also enjoyed an expensive lifestyle. Many workers that were also affected were office staff who did not earn as much, but they lost their jobs too. Loss of job means loss of role, loss of status. And this can have an impact on one's self-image and self-esteem. It also affects the rest of the family.

All these life events can affect human growth and development. If we have unexpected negative events happening to us, this can affect our view of ourselves (self-image) and how we feel about ourselves (self-esteem). On the other hand, negative experiences can be a basis for developing new skills and developing abilities we never knew we had.

Care values commonly used in practitioner work

We have already seen in Chapter 2 how care practitioners promote care values through their work.

The values and standards of care workers is laid down by The Nursing and Midwifery Council (NMC) for nurses (see pages 124–5 in Chapter 2) and by the General Social Care Council for workers in social care (see page 118 in Chapter 2).

Let us look at another section of the guidance from the General Social Care Council.

> **'As a social care worker you must respect the rights of service users while seeking to ensure that their behaviour does not harm themselves or other people.**
> **This includes:**
> - recognising that service users have the right to take risks and helping them to identify and manage potential and actual risks to themselves and others
> - following risk assessment policies and procedures to assess whether the behaviour of service users presents a risk of harm to themselves or to others
> - taking necessary steps to minimise the risks of service users from doing actual or potential harm to themselves or others
> - ensuring that relevant colleagues and agencies are informed about the outcomes and implications of risk assessments'

In many aspects of social care the social care worker has to have a balance between recognising that service users have the right to take risks. The social care worker should help the service user to identify potential and actual risks to themselves and others.

CASE STUDY 7

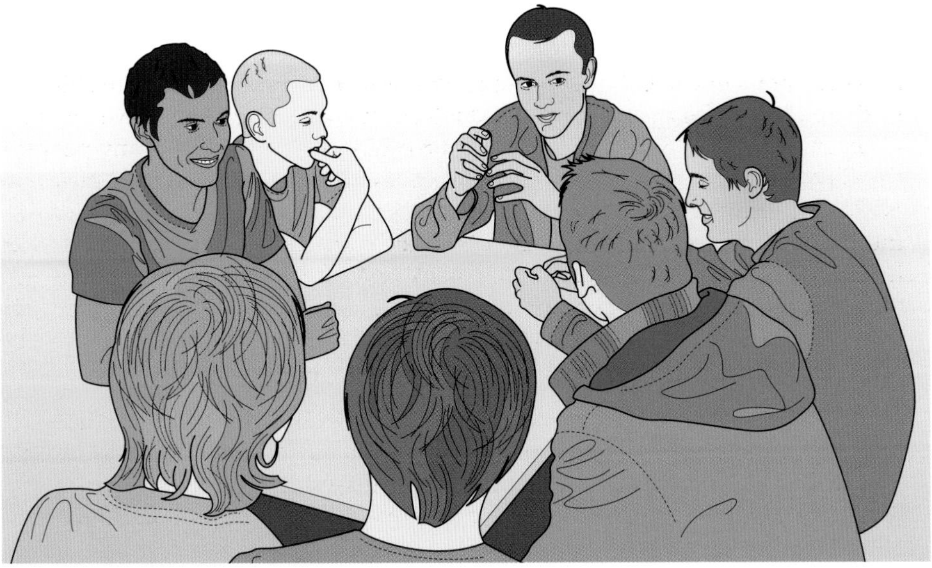

Figure 4.15 Green Gates

Green Gates is a small privately run home for seven young men with learning difficulties and challenging behaviour. The residents of the home have regular meetings with the staff, when they discuss how they want the home organised including the daily menu, outings and leisure activities. Attached

(continued)

CASE STUDY 7 – (continued)

to the home is a small self-contained flat where a client can be prepared for living a more independent life in the community. When one of the young men is given a trial period in the flat, every aspect of the support that will be given is discussed and agreed with the care manager. Brian was given a trial in the flat on the understanding that he would get up on his own in the morning and go to his job in town. He would do all his own shopping, washing and cleaning. Brian agreed to this arrangement. After two weeks in the flat Brian was not getting up and going to work. He lost his job as a result. He was threatening and rude to staff and the flat was dirty.

Look at this case study. If you were the manager of the home, how would you deal with this?

This example shows the problems that may be faced by staff who try to promote independence in their clients. Some clients may find it hard to adjust to being more independent and the staff must decide what strategy to use. The manager decided that Brian had not kept to the agreement and therefore he returned to a room in the main house and another resident was given the flat.

Very often people say they want to go into social care work because they want to help others, but helping people too much can make them dependent on staff. You may feel that Brian should have been helped more. The manager should have got him up in the mornings and made sure he went to work. Brian travelled by public transport.

Care workers have to do a risk assessment to identify how great the risk is for the client and others.

CASE STUDY 8

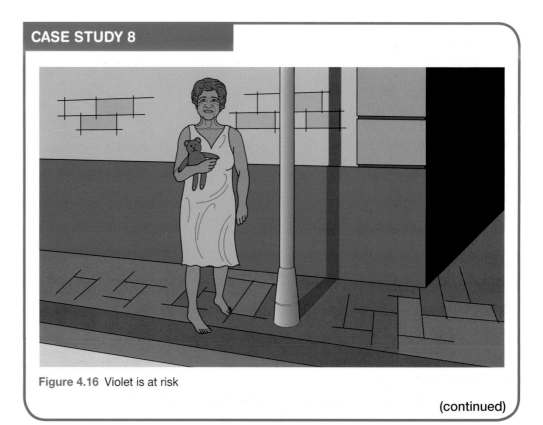

Figure 4.16 Violet is at risk

(continued)

CASE STUDY 8 – (continued)

Violet is a widow who is 84 years old and lives on her own. She has lived in the same house for 60 years. There is limited heating. The bathroom is upstairs so Violet tends to use the outside toilet, so she does not have to climb the stairs. Violet has been diagnosed with Alzheimer's Disease and she was registered as partially sighted 10 years ago. Violet's daughter visits regularly but she lives an hour's drive away. Violet is sometimes very confused and neighbours have contacted social services and the police on numerous occasions, as she often wanders about at night in her nightdress. Recently, she was burgled as she let someone in the house because she thought she recognised him.

Social services organised a care assistant who comes to the house three times a week, to help Vi with cooking, cleaning, the laundry and shopping, but sometimes Vi won't let her into the house. Vi's social worker has a duty of care for Vi's general health and safety. She has met Vi and her daughter to discuss her future care. Vi could be injured or put others at risk if she continue to live at home.

DISCUSSION

Bearing in mind the principles of promoting independence, what could be the best solution for Vi's care?

If she stays at home (which she wants to do) how could she be supported?

What may be the problems if Vi goes into a care home? Remember older people can become very confused if they are moved from familiar surroundings.

Risk assessment

We can see from both these case studies that there are risks involved in the management of care of many client groups. It is the duty of the professional care worker to assess the risks of following a particular course of action. If Vi stays at home, she may have a serious accident or be at risk from abuse or attack. The social worker has to weigh up the advantages and disadvantages of leaving Vi where she is, or of moving her.

In Brian's case, if the manager moves him back into the house, Brian's behaviour may get worse and he could hurt other people in the home. Brian only got the job in the supermarket after a careful risk assessment was made. He first went to the supermarket with a care worker and then he gradually spent more time unaccompanied, getting the bus on his own and working on his own. As Brian is working with the general public, he has to be supervised by one of the store managers so that no member of the public is put at risk.

Care workers have to be very careful when planning activities for teenagers and other young adults. They may want to go to pubs and cinemas. If they go on their own they may be at risk of attack or abuse, but they cannot always be accompanied by a member of staff if they are going to become more independent.

However, some client groups are unable to become fully independent because of their illness or disability.

In our everyday lives we all take risks. We may decide to do a parachute jump, go skiing or travel home late on our own. Usually, when we decide to do an activity like this, we weigh up the problems that may occur and this will influence our decision. In community care, risks of allowing certain activities are also assessed. We may hurt ourselves or others by our actions. When care professionals carry out risk assessments they may be dealing with clients with a range of problems, such as mental distress or learning disabilities, and their behaviour could have consequences for themselves as well as for others.

How care workers promote care values through their work

All health, social care and early years practitioners who work in health and care settings abide by the codes of practice laid down by their professional bodies. For example, the NMC (Nursing and Midwifery Council) states that '... the essence of nursing care is getting to know people as individuals, finding out how they want to be cared for. Health and social care workers should provide care that ensures that respect, dignity and fairness are maintained. These principles apply to all workers in health and social care, including health care assistants, social care workers and other staff.' Further details of the nursing code of care can be found on the website www.nmc-uk.org.

The effects and consequences of these care values not being implemented

We can see from the two case studies above that the social care workers in each case tried to manage the care of their clients, according to the values upheld by their professional body. If care values are not followed, through bad practice, this can have a negative effect on both the care worker and the service user.

EXAMPLE

A senior care practitioner who is working in a care home, has the attitude that the residents are a nuisance. She does not take the trouble to talk to them or their relatives. She does everything as quickly as possible just to get it out of the way – including giving out medication. This attitude will affect the

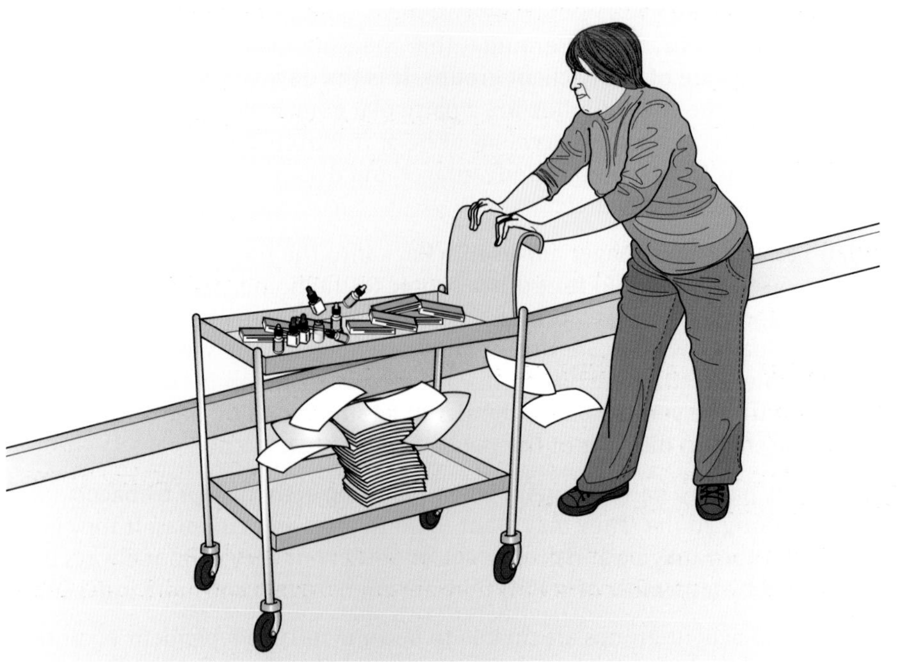

Figure 4.17 A professional approach is essential at all times

(continued)

EXAMPLE – (continued)

behaviour of the rest of the staff so that you get a culture of lack of interest in the residents and a slap-dash attitude to the work. Mistakes may be made when caring for clients – including their medication – so this will have a negative effect on the clients as well. The residents will pick up on the attitudes and behaviour of the staff. Residents will feel that they are a nuisance and will not ask for help when they need it. This may result in residents having falls, as they don't like to ask for help. Their general health will be affected, as staff cannot be bothered to take them out for walks, encourage hobbies and activities.

The care worker may become sloppy and careless in their behaviour and their management of clients in their care. Sometimes this attitude can affect the whole ward or home where the care worker is in.

We can see from this example that it is essential that care staff promote care values in all aspects of their work with clients.

The effects of care values not being followed can be as follows:
For the practitioner:

- will affect their level of job satisfaction
- will see care work as 'just a job'
- poor practice will continue.

For the client:

- will feel undervalued and worthless
- self-esteem will be reduced
- will receive poor care.

Consequences of care values not being followed could be as follows:
For the professional:

- may lose their job
- may be reported to their employer or to their professional body
- may be removed from their professional register.

For the client:

- will lose faith in professional care workers
- recovery may be slow as they may be at risk from infections, illness, injury and even death.

Promoting anti-discriminatory practice

Anti-discriminatory practice is what underpins the work in care settings. Care workers must work with service users in an anti-discriminatory way. We have already looked at this issue in Chapter 2 (page 114). Anti-discrimination means working to eliminate discrimination.

Discrimination means treating people less favourably because they have a personal aspect over which they have no control, i.e. gender, ethnicity, disability, or age.

For example, if only Christian festivals are celebrated at a care home which has Islamic members; or menus for the week don't take account of the dietary needs of certain religious groups.

Discrimination can also be on the basis of age.

Age discrimination occurs in many hospitals.

EXAMPLE

In a hospital in South London anyone who is admitted from A & E will be allocated a bed in the geriatric unit if they are over 75.

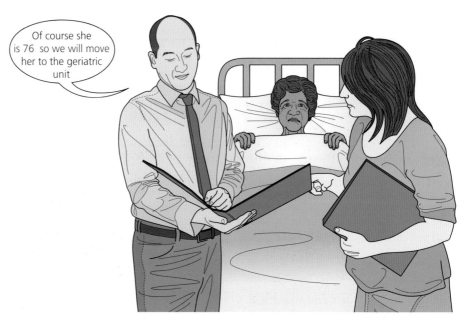

Figure 4.18

As you may know from your own experience there may be a big difference in the levels of health and mobility among people of a certain age. Patients should be allocated a bed according to their clinical need, not because of their age,

We have already discussed individual rights in Chapter 2 (pages 114–15). Rights of the individual may be protected by law, such as the Human Rights Act 1998 (see pages 116–17), or by rights under Charters and Guidelines (see pages 114–15) or are basic human rights.

Discrimination against people with disabilities

Discrimination can include abuse and name calling, for example using terms such as 'spasso' (after spastic). The Spastics Society changed its name to SCOPE because of the problems experienced by people being called 'spastics'. People with a disability can be very vulnerable to abuse as they may be unable to physically defend themselves, or realise they are being made fun of.

Discrimination against people with mental health problems

This can include name calling such as 'loony', 'mental', etc. Many people fear people with mental health problems. Before the 1990 NHS Community Care Act 1990, they were kept in long-stay hospitals distanced from the community. Now there are homes for people with mental health problems in the community, but this group of people are still feared, although they are more likely to hurt themselves than to harm others.

Discrimination against people with a learning disability

This group is also likely to suffer verbal and physical abuse. Many people with learning disabilities are now in the community and may undertake simple jobs in supermarkets, moving trolleys or in cleaning and catering.

All these three groups are entitled to the same rights as the rest of the community. Care workers must ensure that the service user is given the same care and can make the same choices as everyone else.

CASE STUDY 9

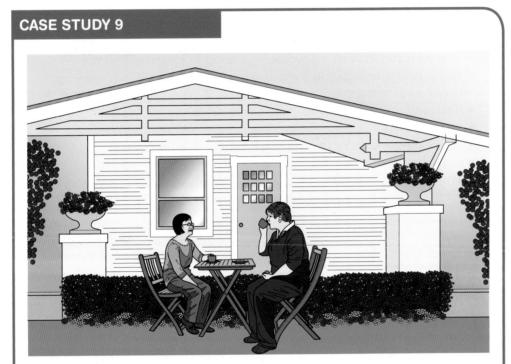

Figure 4.19 Vera in the garden in her home

Vera (66) lives in a bungalow that was built in the grounds of the old long-stay hospital for people with learning disabilities, where she spent most of her life. When government policy approved the closure of all long-stay hospitals for people with learning disabilities, Vera moved into the bungalow with three other women from the hospital that she knew. Vera cannot work now. She used to work in the hospital laundry. She enjoyed it there, but she was never paid for her work. The hospital held discos every Saturday that she enjoyed. Vera has a key worker who visits the bungalow each day and makes sure the residents are well and she gives them their medication. The hospital is quite isolated from the town. They take a minibus each week to the shops, but Vera is getting used to travelling to town on the bus. She has gone with a volunteer several times and soon she will try the journey on her own. She loves her bedroom. She chose the curtains and furniture in it. When she was in the hospital she was in a 30-bedded ward and there was no privacy. The women help choose the menus for each week and they help in the kitchen. They get their own breakfast and snacks and Vera really enjoys this.

Promoting individuals rights to dignity, independence, health and safety

How to maintain a service user's dignity

As carers we need to make sure that we treat the service users we look after with respect at all times.

In June 2008 Ivan Lewis MP Minister for Care Services talked about 'putting dignity at the heart of the care services'. He was talking about the Dignity Challenge. This document states that high quality services that respect people's dignity should at all times:

- have a zero tolerance of all forms of abuse
- support people with the same respect you would want for yourself or a member of your family
- treat each person as an individual by offering a personalised service
- enable people to maintain the maximum possible level of independence, choice and control
- listen and support people to express their needs and wants
- respect people's right to privacy
- ensure people feel able to complain without fear of retribution
- engage with family members and carers as care partners
- assist people to maintain confidence and a positive self-esteem
- act to alleviate people's loneliness and isolation.

Ivan Lewis asked people to put themselves forward as Dignity Champions.

CASE STUDY 10 –This is Doris' story

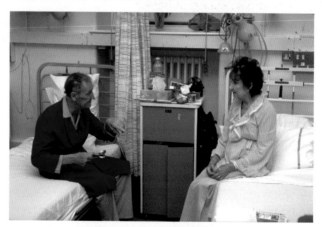

Figure 4.20 Mixed-sex wards do not give patients the dignity they should have

I am 77 and I fell and broke my hip. I had the operation and then I was put in a mixed-sex ward. I felt dreadful. The only man who has ever seen me in a nightie was my husband. There are a lot of old men in here. They wander about going to the toilet in the night time. I feel embarrassed using the bedpan or commode, as the curtains don't really give you any privacy. I was really upset last week when some poor woman died and there was no privacy for the family. If you cannot die in dignity I think that is awful. I hope I die at home.

One of the key problems in hospitals in meeting this challenge has been the continuing use of mixed-sex wards.

There is a policy across the NHS to reduce all mixed-sex wards and, if possible, to get rid of them altogether. Mixed-sex wards are also a problem in mental health trusts, where there have been examples of male patients attacking female patients.

Dignity

Treating a patient with dignity includes calling a patient by their preferred name. Older people may not want to be called by their first name. Some carers call their clients 'dear' and 'love' which is seen as unhelpful. Guidelines will be issued in 2009 by the Nursing and Midwifery Council about how nurses should speak to people in their care.

The dignity of patients in hospital is assured by the Health Care Commission. You can find details of reports made on hospital trusts and PCTs on the health care commission website www.healthcarecommission.org.uk

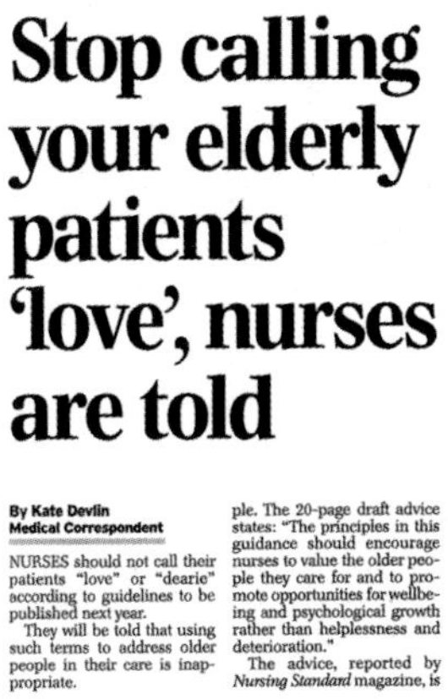

Health and Safety

As we saw in Chapter 2, health and safety is very important in all services provided by health, social care and early years services.

Accidents at work

Although every care is taken when looking after people, accidents will happen. Falls are a real problem whether you are looking at safety issues in a playground, in a residential home or in a hospital. Most hospitals have a falls policy. When anyone over 50-years-of age is admitted to hospital, either as routine or via Accident and Emergency, they are assessed to see whether they have a history of falls; if they have dizzy spells, or they are on medication which can make them giddy. In order to reduce the risk of further falls, patients may be kept in a bed near the nurses' station so they can keep an eye on them.

Falls affecting babies and young children

All children fall but there are ways of ensuring they do not fall too far, or are hurt. If you are working in a nursery or infants class, there will be regulations about how to protect the children in your care:

Stop calling your elderly patients 'love', nurses are told

By Kate Devlin
Medical Correspondent

NURSES should not call their patients "love" or "dearie" according to guidelines to be published next year.

They will be told that using such terms to address older people in their care is inappropriate.

ple. The 20-page draft advice states: "The principles in this guidance should encourage nurses to value the older people they care for and to promote opportunities for wellbeing and psychological growth rather than helplessness and deterioration."

The advice, reported by *Nursing Standard* magazine, is

Figure 4.21 Care workers should be careful to call patients by their chosen name

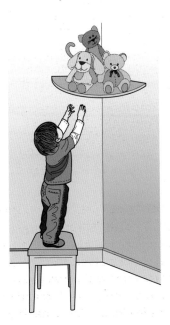

Figure 4.22 Children are at risk of falls

- babies should never be left unattended on a table work surface, bed or sofa; lie them on the floor instead
- stair gates are an essential piece of equipment at the bottom and top of stairs as well as across a doorway
- vertical bars should be fitted to dangerous windows (horizontal bars encourage climbing)
- fit child-proof window safety catches to all windows
- use a harness in the highchair, pram pushchair or supermarket trolley
- teach children how to use stairs safely, teach them to come downstairs backwards on all fours
- do not place furniture under windows where children may be encouraged to climb.

If you take children out to the park or playground, you need to ensure they are safe but encourage them to take part in active play.

Interpersonal skills

These are skills we use in everyday life when we relate to other people through communication.

Health and social care workers need good interpersonal skills. We have already looked at the skills and qualities needed by health and social care workers on page 104.

We will now focus on communication skills.

Promoting effective communication and relationships

The health and social care worker must be able to communicate effectively with a wide range of patients, clients and other workers:

- babies/children
- adolescents
- young adults
- older people
- other health workers
- doctors
- nurses
- teachers
- police
- social workers.

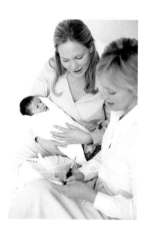

Figure 4.23 Care workers have to be able to communicate well with all groups of patients

Lack of effective communication between the care worker and the patient will mean that the client may not receive the support they need.

Communication can take many forms. In this section we will be looking at communication in the form of:

- verbal communication
- non-verbal communication
- written communication.

Verbal communication

Everyone says they know how to talk, but in health and social care it is important to use verbal communication effectively when:

- assessing patients
- identifying needs
- giving information
- encouraging patients to express their own views and be independent.

Questions

Most health and social workers use questions every day.

There are several types of question.

1. **Closed questions**, for example: How old are you? What is your name? Are you married?
   These questions are appropriate when brief factual material is needed, but they do not encourage conversation and expression of thoughts and feelings.
2. **Open (or open-ended) questions**. These give an opportunity for fuller, deeper answers, for example: How do you feel about moving into sheltered housing? Is there anything you need to know about how to breast feed the baby? How, what, feel and think are useful words for encouraging a full response.
3. **Biased questions**. These indicate the answer the questioner wants or expects to hear, for example: 'You have settled into the routine of the home, haven't you?' 'It isn't necessary to go over your medication again, is it?'
4. **Multiple questions**. These include more than one question and can cause confusion, for example, 'Is this a serious problem, when did it start?' 'How did the accident happen, what did you do?'

It is the responsibility of the health and social care worker to make sure that communication is effective.

Barriers to communication

Communication is a two-way process. We all communicate every day. Think about a typical day in your life and the communications that take place.

You may have identified some of the following:

- informal conversation with friends, either one to one or else in a group
- more formal discussions at work or college
- telephone conversations, formal and informal
- letters from friends, emails, faxes.

All these forms of communication use words, either spoken or written.

Think about a recent communication that went well. Why did it go well?

Now think about a recent communication that left you feeling awkward, angry, or frustrated. What was the problem?

Barriers to communication can include the following:

- insufficient information is given
- the environment is unhelpful – noisy, lack of privacy, too many people talking at the same time
- the other person does not seem interested in what you have to say
- lack of understanding due to language used.

Listening skills

Listening skills are very important in health and social care. In ordinary conversations there tends to be a pattern to conversation; for example, Mary tells Surinder about what she did on Saturday night, and Surinder tells Mary what she did on Saturday night. We can see that there is an exchange of information. In effective listening the pattern is different. In effective listening you need to concentrate on the feelings of the other person and put your own views and feelings to one side.

Look at the following conversation:

> **EXAMPLE**
>
> *Jane*: I feel very tired. I suppose it is my age; everything seems to be such an effort.
>
> *Practice nurse*: Yes, the "change" is no fun is it? I have awful night sweats and shout at the family.

What is the problem with the practice nurse's response?

You can see that the nurse is more concerned with expressing her own feelings, rather than listening effectively to Jane.

Listening effectively can be developed through the method called **reflecting back**. The care worker checks that they fully understand what the client is saying by restating what has been said. This helps the client to make their feelings clear. Reflecting back is used only in the discussion of feelings, not in other situations.

Read this example of reflecting back:

> **EXAMPLE**
>
> *Mother*: I just feel so useless. I never realised having a baby was such hard work. I seem to run about all day and I never get the place straight, and I feel so tired.
>
> *Health Visitor*: Why do you think you feel so tired?
>
> *Mother*: I suppose I feel I want everything to be perfect. My mother-in-law lives nearby. She is always popping in. Her house always looks perfect. She must think I am useless.
>
> *Health Visitor*: Why do you think your mother-in-law thinks you are useless?
>
> *Mother*: She has never approved of me, and it is even worse now.
>
> *Health Visitor*: Do you think it has got worse since you had the baby?

By reflecting back in this way, the health worker may be able to help the patient identify the real problem. In this case, the problem may be the relationship between the two women rather than the birth of the baby. On the other hand, it could be that the mother has post-natal depression. In either case, effective listening is a useful tool in helping people to understand their feelings.

You may also meet people who have specific difficulties in communication.

People who have visual impairment

When you meet a client with visual problems it is very important that you introduce yourself by name and what you do. You also need to explain carefully what you are doing, for example:

- giving an injection or medication
- changing a dressing
- taking them to another department.

If the person is able to walk, you need to ask them if they want to hold on to you. Don't just grab them by the arm and rush them off!

People with a hearing problem

You need to ask them what will help them to hear you well. They may be able to lip read, so you will need to:

- stand or sit in front of them
- speak at your normal pace
- don't cover your mouth or chew gum, as this makes it difficult to lip read
- don't stand with your face away from them while you talk.

If someone has one-sided deafness, make sure you are talking to them on their 'good side'.

If they use hearing aids, make sure the battery is working and they are turned on.

Maintaining confidentiality of information

Confidentiality is a key part of daily work in health, social care and early years services. As we saw in Chapter 2 it is important that service users can trust care workers. Chatting about your work and the service users you care for is so easy to do. Apart from breaking confidentiality about clients to friends and family, it is easy to talk about clients to other clients.

EXAMPLE 1

Brenda works in a nursing home for 28 residents. There is a lot of sickness at the moment and Brenda is feeling the strain of rushing about trying to get all the work done. She rushes into Mrs Baker's room (without knocking first).

Brenda: Hello dear how are you? Shall I run the bath for you and you can freshen up? Sorry, I am a bit late but Sally is off sick and Mrs Davies had a little accident – not her fault, the poor old dear – but I had to sort her out before I could come to you.

Mrs Baker: Oh dear.

DISCUSSION

What do you think of this scenario? You may have made various comments about Brenda, for example:

- She did not knock before entering the room.
- She called Mrs Baker 'dear'.
- She talked about another resident's problems to Mrs Baker.
- Mrs Baker probably thinks that Brenda will discuss her private matters with other people.

There are a many situations when it is necessary to preserve confidentiality. For example, in the following situations.

- A child at the nursery school is HIV positive – a parent asks you if there is anything wrong with him.
- A patient has an AIDs related chest infection – his mother wants to know the details.
- In your work on the genito-urinary unit you see a neighbour who is attending for an STI test (sexually transmitted infection).

- You work on the assisted conception unit and a patient tells you they are considering using a sperm donor because her husband has a low sperm count.
- You are working in reception at the doctor's surgery and someone rings up and wants to know the results of her blood test.

There are rules – sometimes called protocols – about how information is given, to whom and by whom. In the case of the doctor's receptionist, the doctor will tell the receptionist what to do. The doctor may ask the patient to speak to him about the results on the phone; if there is a problem about the results the patient would be asked to make an appointment. Receptionists in surgeries and in schools must respect confidentiality at all time. They may overhear conversations about service users, but they should keep the information to themselves. These are the basic rules about giving information:

- You should only give information with consent
- You should only give information on a 'need to know' basis – for example if a child at nursery school has asthma or diabetes, staff need to know so that they can look after the child properly.
- You only give information that is needed. You don't want to be told everything – we know people like this ourselves. We ask them where they bought a dress and they give us a long story when we just need the name of the shop!
- You must always check the identity of the person you are speaking to – this is especially important in a hospital where someone may ring up and ask how someone is. Why do they need to know and who are they? In cases of domestic abuse or other problematic cases, you need to be very careful. It may seem hard to be suspicious of people, but your role is to protect the patient from possible harm.
- Only give limited information. It may be irritating for relatives to be told that their mother is comfortable, but if they want more details they can contact senior staff or visit the hospital.

Acknowledging individual personal beliefs and identity

Care workers in health, social care and early years services work with a range of people who may have personal beliefs that are very important to them. Religious practices can have an impact on the way service users wish to be supported. As a direct carer, you should support services users when they make choices about:

- diet
- pregnancy
- childbirth
- who should care for them
- clothing worn
- care of infants and children
- care of older people
- care for the dying.

You should not force your own religious beliefs on clients and you must respect their beliefs. Nowadays, the UK is a multi-cultural society, but in the 20th century professionals had to learn about the beliefs and practices of their clients. There were many examples of professionals not understanding why some minority groups behaved the way they did.

The diets of certain ethnic groups based on religious grounds were not acknowledged As care workers, we need to be aware of the taboos of certain foods as well as the significance of fasting. As care workers, we should be aware of the main issues about diets.

These are some of the main diets we need to be aware of:

Hinduism – orthodox Hindus are not allowed to eat any animal, particularly the cow. Milk is acceptable.

Islam – neither pork nor any other pig products may be eaten. The only meat that is allowed is from animals with a cloven hoof (like beef and lamb), but this meat must be prepared by a halal butcher.

Judaism – as with Islam, pork and other pig products are not allowed. Only kosher meat is allowed. Meat and milk dishes are never mixed in the same meal.

Sikhism – beef is strictly forbidden, but pork is allowed and meat must be slaughtered in a special way, it is important that care workers respect the religious views of all service users.

There are rituals related to pregnancy and childbirth and to death and dying.

Jehovah's witnesses are allowed to accept blood transfusions although some choose not to because they believe that blood transfusions are not allowed according to the Bible.

CASE STUDY 12

A young woman was brought into hospital. She was having a baby, but the placenta had become detached and she had heavy bleeding. The surgeons wanted to operate quickly to save her life and that of her baby. Her husband explained to the surgeon that they were Jehovah's witnesses and they would not allow a blood transfusion. The surgeon explained to the couple that if they did not give a transfusion the woman could die and so could the baby. The women said it was God's will. Both she and the baby died.

In these situations, the care professional must explain in detail what would happen if the treatment was not given. The couple were told about the possible outcome if a transfusion was not given, but they still refused.

As care workers, we have to support service users in their decisions.

How these care values are reflected through practitioner interaction with service users in their attitudes and behaviour, and through professional training and development of care practitioners

In this section, we have seen several examples of practitioner interaction with service users. It is essential that the attitudes and behaviour of care workers reflect the care values. Very often, behaviour that is not helpful to service users is thoughtless rather than deliberately negative.

Here are some examples of the behaviour of care workers. Think about why they behave like this and what might help them think more carefully in future.

1. Two nurses are making the bed while Mary (25) is lying in it. They roll her from side to side while they change the bottom sheet. They talk to each other about their plans for the weekend.

2. The practice nurse is immunising a large number of people who have come for their flu jab. She asks each patient for their name, checks their name on the record sheet and gives them an injection.

3. Jane (55) has come to the outpatients for the results of a brain scan. She is quite nervous. The doctor tells her the scan shows that Jane has a small brain tumour. She tells Jane she will refer her to a specialist hospital. Jane asks her what the scan showed. The doctor says she hasn't seen the scan herself; she just has the report.

4. Merya is expecting her second baby. Her first baby died at 17-days-old from a cot death. Merya is very worried that something is wrong with this baby. The midwife tells Merya that everything seems fine. Merya says she is worried because of what happened to her first baby. The midwife asked her what happened. When Merya tells her, the midwife asks her if she breastfed the baby. Merya says she tried but she could not manage it. The midwife then says, 'Oh, if you breastfed the first baby that would not have happened'. Merya is now terrified that she will not be able to breastfeed the second baby and she feels guilty about her first daughter.

5. Two student nurses are tidying up the bed of Thomas (35) who had a stroke. Thomas can hear but he cannot speak. The student nurses complain about the mess he has made in the bed.

Let's go through each example in turn.

1. The two nurses are showing lack of respect for the patient by ignoring her while they make the bed. Perhaps they need to have some training in how to use their communication skills.

2. The practice nurse is probably focusing on the large number of people she has to immunise in the clinic. She feels it is more important to make sure of the names of the people she is treating, than to talk to people and put them at their ease. She is under pressure so perhaps this is the result of bad planning, when an extra nurse could have shared the work load.

3. The doctor seems to have little understanding about the anxiety Jane must be feeling. Care workers should always read the patient notes carefully. In this case, the doctor should have seen the scan before she saw Jane. It is always important in care services that you have all the information you need, so you can reassure the patient.

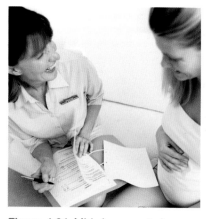

Figure 4.24 Midwives must always be supportive

4. Pregnant women are often very anxious and in Merya's case her anxiety is understandable. The midwife should have read the notes carefully. Cot death is something that all mothers fear and because Merya has had this experience, she will be even more anxious. The midwife should reassure and support Merya. By expressing her views that Merya was at fault in her baby's death by not breastfeeding the child, she has caused Merya a great deal of anxiety. Midwives must always be supportive to the mothers in their care.

5. Care workers often make the mistake that if someone is unable to speak they cannot hear. Perhaps they need training on strokes and stroke care. They seem to be lacking an understanding of their patient's needs.

Most professionals now have to have Continuing Professional Development (CPD) when they have to undergo training if they are to retain their professional qualification. All doctors have to show they have attended training events and updated their knowledge. In one PCT, the GPs videoed some of their consultations with patients and these films were discussed with the GP's mentor to discuss how their practice could be improved. The patients were asked for their consent and they really enjoyed the experience. Videos were not taken of physical examinations.

All workers in health and social care have to have regular training to update their knowledge and practice in certain aspects of their work. This may vary according to the role of the worker, but all workers have to have training to update them on:

- safeguarding clients from abuse
- first aid, including resuscitation techniques
- manual handling – how to lift and move patients and equipment.

The consequences that may arise if service practitioners have not effectively implemented care values

The possibility of discrimination

We have seen in this book that certain groups are more likely to experience discrimination, for example:

- ethnic minorities
- older people
- people with disabilities
- people with learning disabilities
- people with mental health problems
- gay or lesbian people
- women.

All care professionals should have training so that they are aware of how certain groups can be discriminated against. As we have seen on page 206, discriminatory language and behaviour should be avoided at all times.

The possibility of social exclusion

Social exclusion refers to the isolation of individuals or groups because they have been rejected by others. This could be because of bullying at school or at work. A wider definition of social exclusion can refer to groups of people who are excluded from society because of a range of factors such as poverty, poor housing, unemployment and poor education. This may affect their access to health care. Older people and people from ethnic minorities are more likely to experience social exclusion, and health and care workers must try to reach these groups.

The effect of poor practice on the self-esteem and self-concept of service users

Direct carers must always deliver services professionally and respect the service user. Some client groups may have difficulty when they see their GP because of hearing difficulties, the medical jargon used and the speed of the consultation. (GPs are allowed 10 minutes for a consultation.) Patients can be made to feel a nuisance if they ask questions and this has a bad effect on the patient's self-esteem. The self-concept of service users is affected by the way care workers behave towards them.

We saw that GPs have recorded their consultations with patients. If you are caring for someone in their own home, in a nursery situation and in a care home, do you think recording your practice might be a helpful way of reminding you about the importance of good practice?

Disempowerment

Empowering someone is about encouraging them and supporting them to be independent and make decisions in their lives. Disempowerment is about controlling people so they do as they are told and cannot make decisions. Look at the following examples and decide if empowerment or disempowerment is taking place.

1. In Rose Cottage residential home, residents are lined up outside the toilets each morning at 10 am after they have had their coffee.
2. In Tadpoles nursery class the children decide whether they want to do sand play or water play.
3. In hospital, patients are woken up at 6 am so that they can be given their medication and have their TPR (temperature, pulse rate and respiration rate) charts updated before the night staff go off duty.
4. In the Beeches home for people with learning disabilities, residents plan and cook the evening meal.

It may be helpful to ask yourself why certain activities such as getting up and going to bed, take place at certain times. Is it to help the service users, or is it to fit round the staff?

Lack of self-worth

Lack of self worth is linked to how we feel about ourselves. If care workers do not respect the people they are supporting, this can make the patient feel useless and a burden.

The development of self-concept and personal relationships

In Chapter 1 we looked at the development of self-concept in great detail. We realise that there are many factors that affect our self-concept, such as age, appearance, gender, social class, ethnicity and culture. Some factors we cannot control, such as the family we are born into and whether we are male or female. We have seen in Chapter 3 that education is linked to economic factors in our lives. In developing our relationships with others we have seen that our experiences in childhood can affect us for the rest of our lives. Our emotional development is very closely linked with our social development. Our sexual orientation can influence our personal development, especially if we are homosexual rather than heterosexual. Our personal development continues throughout our life course and the experiences we have during our lives make us who we are. It is important to understand why people behave the way they do; and also that older people were once young; disabled people may not have always been limited; people with depression and other mental health needs may not have always had these problems. We should treat all our clients as we would like to be treated ourselves.

CASE STUDY 13 – Lucy

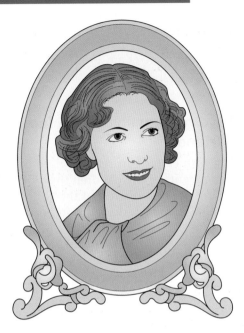

Figure 4.25 Edna as a young woman

Lucy was doing her work experience in a residential home for older people. She was annoyed that she could not have been placed in a nursery, which is what she wanted. She complained to her friends about the old people; they were so slow; they took ages to walk about; they had problems hearing her and some of them were very confused. One morning she was in the room of Edna, a resident, and she noticed a photograph of a beautiful young girl of about 18, or so. She asked who the girl was. Edna said 'that was me before I met my husband and got married'. Lucy suddenly realised that these old people that she complained about had all been young. They had relationships and experiences like everyone else. She found out that some of the residents had been very successful in their careers. The more she talked to them, the more she realised that her initial reaction had been discriminatory and unfair.

Relationship building with service users

Just as Lucy realised Edna and the other residents had stories to tell and she was able to see beyond the stereotype of older people, so care practitioners must build relationships with the service users in their care. This may be difficult if you are working in a busy hospital ward, where people come in and go out very rapidly. It is easier if you are working in a nursery, care home or looking after a client in their home. We all know that we feel better about ourselves if someone takes an interest in us and treats us with respect. Obviously, we are all human and we may like some people more than others, but we should try to build a relationship with the people we come into contact with in our work.

Empowerment of service users

We have discussed how we can empower service users by encouraging them to make decisions about their care as well as other aspects of their lives, which may include going out to the pub or going out for the day. The new government policy of **Transforming Social Care** will give more power and control to service users of the care they receive. Once they are assessed by social services, individuals will be given an individual budget to spend as they wish on the care they need. Before this change, the care needs of a person were assessed by social services and a care package developed and chosen by the care manager. Many government policies are about improving patient's choice and empowering service users in all aspects of health, social care and early years services.

Promoting positive relationships with family, partners, colleagues and friends

Care workers working with early years services need to develop positive relationships with the parents of the children they look after. Both sides have an interest in promoting the best interest of the child. If there is a named nurse or lead professional involved, this is an important relationship to develop.

Care workers do not work in isolation. They will be working in partnership with other professionals – as part of a multi-disciplinary team. It important these relationships work well in order to develop an integrated approach for the service user. Some service users may be quite isolated from friends and family – others may have a lot of family and friends. It is important that these family members are aware of the care worker who is responsible for supporting their mother/father so that they can discuss any problems with them.

Promoting and supporting health improvement

Chapters 2 and 3 covered factors affecting health and well-being throughout the life course and the effects of these factors on the individual's health and well-being.

Different ways health professionals can support service users to change their lifestyles in order to improve health

Diet

(See the sections on *'Diet'*, in Chapter 1, page 23 and Chapter 3, page 137, that explain the positive and negative influences of nutrition on health and well-being.)

If it is suspected that a client does not have a healthy diet, a health professional, such as a GP or health visitor, may refer them to a **Registered Dietician** (RD). The dietician will assess their diet. Practical guidance will then be given using up-to-date public health and scientific research on food and health. This guidance will help the client make appropriate lifestyle and food choices. Recently changes have been made, so that a person can refer themselves to an NHS dietician without the need to see another health professional first.

Regular exercise

(See the sections on 'Exercise' in Chapter 1, page 24 and Chapter 3, page 140, explain the influence of physical activity and lack of physical activity on health and well-being.)

A health professional, such as a GP or practice nurse, may prescribe exercise to a patient who they think needs to be more active (see Figure 4.26). They will refer them to a facility such as a leisure centre or gym for a supervised exercise programme. Swimming, aerobics, yoga and weight training are examples of the types of exercise that may be undertaken.

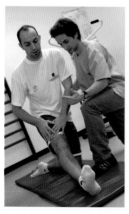

Figure 4.26 Exercise may be prescribed to some patients

Patients who are specifically targeted include those who have:

- coronary heart disease
- high blood pressure
- obesity
- diabetes
- mental health problems, including depression
- musculo-skeletal problems, such as chronic back pain.

Supportive relationships

(See the sections on *'Family'* and *'Friends'* in Chapter 1, pages 26 and 43 and Chapter 3, page 148.)

Health professionals recognise the importance of supportive relationships in improving a person's health (see Figure 4.27).

For this reason, they may encourage friends or relatives who are carers to take advantage of the help and support available. This may include the provision of:

- help in the home (for example, with cooking or personal care, such as washing and dressing of the person cared for)
- day care of the person cared for, to give the carer a break
- equipment that will give the carer piece of mind, such as a mobile phone
- carers services, such as counselling or alternative therapies for the carersupport groups for carers
- training opportunities, for example in lifting, first aid, or stress reduction.

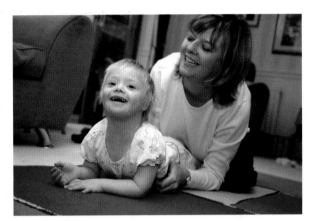

Figure 4.27 Health professionals recognise the importance of supportive relationships

ACTIVITY

Find out what help and support is available specifically for young carers.

Work

(See the sections on *'Employment/unemployment'* and *'Employment status'* in Chapter 1, pages 32 and 27 and Chapter 3, pages 150–1 and 155 which explain the importance of work in maintaining good health.)

Health professionals are aware of the importance of employment in helping all aspects of a person's health and well-being. It is thought that work can have therapeutic benefits, particularly for people suffering from stress and mental illness. The longer a person is off work, statistically, the less likely they are to return to employment. Some people have criticised the benefits system, suggesting that the incapacity benefit paid to sick and disabled people, makes them less likely to work, and that this has an adverse effect on their health.

In recognition of the positive effects of work, there are many examples of patients being encouraged to remain in, or seek, employment where possible. The example of back pain, below, illustrates this.

Back pain

Figure 4.28, below, illustrates how physical and psychological factors can combine to give two interrelated vicious circles that interconnect to increase or prolong back pain.

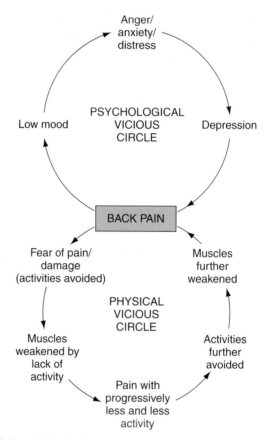

Figure 4.28 The 'vicious circles' of back pain

In order to help break or prevent the cycle, health professionals recommend that people with back pain are encouraged to stay in work, or get back to work as soon as possible and, if necessary, negotiate with their employer less physically strenuous duties. If necessary, a local Disability Employment Adviser can arrange work assessment and retraining and also provide equipment that would help with getting back to work.

Rest and sleep

'Sufficient sleep is not a luxury – it is a necessity – and should be thought of as a vital sign of good health.'

Why do we need to sleep?

Sleep is important for both physical and mental functioning and well-being. Scientists are still not able to agree exactly why we need to sleep, but the following reasons are thought to be important:

- It gives a **chance for the body to recover** from the day's activities.
- It is important for **brain development**.
- Important **chemicals and hormones are released** during sleep.

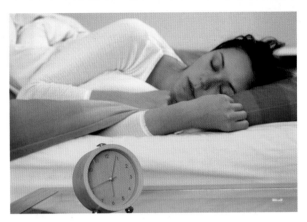

Figure 4.29 Sufficient sleep is an essential aspect of health promotion

Short term effects of lack of sleep

Most people have had the experience of not having enough sleep at night, and then noticing that they don't feel or perform at their best the following day. Lack of sleep can cause accidents because brain function is affected. Without enough sleep, the following are affected:

- concentration span
- language
- planning
- memory
- sense of time
- judgement
- ability to sense the feelings of others.

It is said that after being awake for 18 hours, a person's performance is decreased by the same amount as drinking two glasses of wine (the drink driving limit). A number of disasters have been blamed, at least partially for lack of sleep. Examples include Chernobyl and the Challenger shuttle explosion.

Long term effects of lack of sleep

There is now evidence that a lack of sleep can also lead to chronic (long term) diseases and conditions such as:

- depression
- diseases of the heart and circulation, such as high blood pressure, heart attack and stroke
- diabetes
- obesity.

How much sleep do we need?

We need enough sleep to make us feel refreshed and to stay awake and alert throughout the day. Table 4.4 shows recommended sleep guidelines for different age groups. As you can see, people need different amounts of sleep at different times of their lives. The amount of sleep needed also varies between individuals of the same age.

Life stage	Age	Hours sleep per night
Infants (will include naps during the day)	Birth-2 months	10.5–18
	2–12 months	14–15
	12–18 months	13–15
	18 months–3 years	12–14
Childhood	3–5 years	11–13
	5–10 years	9–11
Adolescence	11–18 years	At least 8.5–9.5
Adults	19–65	Typically 7–9
Later adulthood	65+	Variable, but typically 5–6 It is likely that there will be: • Frequent waking through the night • Loss of deepest levels of sleep • More daytime napping • Earlier bedtimes and wake-up

Data from the National Sleep Foundation

Table 4.4 How much sleep do you need?

How to get a good night's sleep

The promotion of good sleeping patterns is sometimes known as 'sleep hygiene'. Health professionals will give advice on how a person who has insomnia can improve their sleep. The following recommendations are made by The Sleep Council:

- Stick to a routine – aim to go to bed and get up at the same time each day.
- Your sleeping environment is important. Your bedroom should be quiet, dark and at the correct temperature.
- Use your bed for sleeping – not for reading, watching television, listening to music or playing electronic games.
- Physical activity during the day may help, but avoid for a few hours before bedtime.
- Avoid heavy meals in the evening.
- Avoid too much alcohol. You may fall asleep, but may wake during the night.
- Avoid caffeine (for example in coke, tea and coffee).
- Make lists to help you deal with any worries that may keep you awake.
- Before you go to bed, relax by taking a warm bath, doing yoga or listening to relaxing music.
- If you can't sleep, don't lie there worrying. Get up, do something relaxing and then go back to bed.

In some cases, a GP may refer a patient to a Sleep Clinic for additional help.

Stress

(See the section on *'Stress'*, in Chapter 3, that explains the effect of stress on health and well-being on pages 163–5.)

Health professionals will encourage those suffering from stress to identify the cause of stress and use positive ways of coping, such as changing work patterns, exercise, the use of relaxation and having adequate rest (see Figure 4.30). They will support them in avoiding methods of coping which are harmful to health, such as using tobacco, alcohol, or illegal drugs.

Managing stress can be divided into four aspects:

- Removing or reducing the source of stress
- Learning to change the way the source of stress is perceived
- Reducing the physical effect of stress
- Learning ways of coping.

Patients with stress may be referred to trained counsellor or psychotherapist for either individual or group help with the development of stress management skills.

Complementary therapies may also be recommended, such as:

- Aromatherapy
- Reflexology
- Meditation
- Yoga
- Alexander technique.

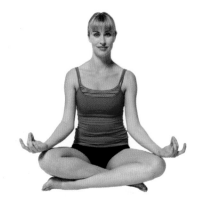

Figure 4.30 Health professionals may encourage the use of relaxation techniques to reduce stress

Usually, medication will not be prescribed, although some types of anxiety can be treated with anti-depressants. It is likely that the health professional will think it preferable to give support in removing the cause of stress and promoting coping techniques.

Recreational activities

Recreational activities, which may include exercise, relaxation, hobbies, cultural activities or just socialising, give many benefits. Depending on the choice of leisure activity, benefits may include:

- A less sedentary life style
- weight loss
- reduction in blood pressure
- lower risk of heart disease
- lower risk of dementia
- less stress
- higher self-esteem.

Many health professionals encourage those they are caring for to participate in recreational activities. This may range from those looking after children in nurseries and schools; those looking after the elderly in a residential or day care setting; and nurses and doctors who need to persuade their patients to exercise more, reduce stress or give up smoking.

ACTIVITY

a) List some of your leisure activities.
b) For each activity, think about which aspects of your health and well-being it contributes to – physical, intellectual, emotional or social.
c) Can you think of other leisure activities you could do, so that all aspects of your health and well-being (physical, intellectual, emotional or social) are addressed?

Financial resources

(See the sections on 'Economic factors' in Chapter 1, pages 30–1 and Chapter 3, page 154, which explain the importance of financial resources in maintaining good health.)

Health professionals have a role in helping people who are living in poverty, such as older people, single parents and people with disabilities. They are likely to see vulnerable people in their own homes, and so are important in identifying clients and patients who are living in poverty. They can then make sure that they have access to programs that are targeted at the less well-off. Without external support, these people may be unlikely to apply for the help available.

Health professionals will also help those in poverty by providing education, for example on how to keep warm or how to have a healthy diet on a low income.

How these factors can influence health

Positive influence

The positive effects of a good diet, regular exercise, the type of work you do, and other lifestyle factors that keep you well, also reduce the likelihood of you becoming ill and will increase your life expectancy. However, positive influences affecting you health are often linked to social and economic factors; this is why we see a difference in morbidity and mortality rates between the upper social classes and the lower social classes, who may experience poverty, poor lousing, poor diet and heavy types of work if they are employed.

Negative influence

On the other hand, those groups who are in poverty, have limited income, poor housing and may have problems related to stress are more likely to experience sickness rates, premature death and poor mental health.

One of the health targets for the UK is to reduce health inequalities between the middle class groups and the lower working classes.

'Choosing Health' is a document published by the Department of Health in 2004.

Read the following excerpt from the document:

'the environment we live in, our social networks, our sense of security, socio-economic circumstances, facilities and resources in our local neighbourhood can affect individual health.

There are unacceptable differences in people's experiences of health between different areas, and between different groups of people within the same area. Action by local authorities working with local communities, businesses and voluntary groups to tackle local health issues makes a difference to the opportunities for both adults and children to choose a healthier lifestyle.'

This makes it clear that the government expect local areas to work together to reduce health inequalities.

In a London borough the Public Health Unit did a survey to see if there were health inequalities in the area.

Three out of four people reported good health in general and two out of three expected to be in good health in the future.

However, the survey showed large socio-demographic difference in health experiences and expectations.

81% of people in higher socio-economic groups consider themselves to be in good health now, compared with 61% of people in the lowest socio-economic groups.

78% of the people in the higher socio-economic groups expected to be in good health in 10 years time, compared to 53% of the lowest socio-economic groups.

The borough has 18 wards (or districts). In the most deprived wards there is significant material deprivation. In these most deprived wards the life expectancy is also lower than elsewhere in the borough. These wards have the:

- highest number of teenage pregnancies
- highest number of people who are unemployed
- highest number of people on benefits as their main source of income
- highest number of ethnic minorities
- highest number of older people over 65.

> **KEY TERM**
>
> **Material deprivation** – the level of poverty in an area, taking into account factors such as employment, education, housing, income, health and well-being and the environment.

The ward has a large council estate that was built in the 1930s. The younger population tends to be continually changing, so it is difficult to feel a sense of community. There is a drugs and alcohol problem. The health profile of this area shows that the rate of early deaths from heart disease and stroke is falling, but this is at a slower rate than in the rest of England. Estimates suggest that 17% of people in the ward have a binge-drinking problem.

Statistics of this borough show there has been an overall improvement in health, but there is still a gap between the different areas – the most deprived and the least deprived. People in deprived areas still have a shorter life expectancy and are more likely to suffer from respiratory and cardiac disease. They are also more likely to suffer mental health problems and have more time unable to work because of ill-health.

It would appear that socio-economic factors are of great importance in health and well-being.

Health promotion

There are a number of different definitions of health promotion, but one which is often used is the WHO (World Health Organisation) definition:

Health promotion is the process of enabling people to increase control over, and to improve, their health.

Health promotion involves providing information to others which will help them to improve their health and well-being. It may include the development of health improvement plans, either for groups or individuals.

The aims of health promotion

Raising awareness

Every health promotion programme has to raise awareness of health issues and the factors affecting health. The process of health education about these issues can be through leaflets, advertisements, focus groups, contacting people at work or at school and in leisure settings. Once you have provided the information, public health workers have to find ways of motivating and persuading people to make changes in their lifestyle for their health. Once people are motivated to make changes, they need to be supported in their choice so that their skills and confidence improve.

Do these approaches work?

CASE STUDY 14

In a local branch of Age Concern there is a project concerned with improving the health and fitness of people over 50. The project manager assesses the person in their home and discusses with them the changes they could make in their lifestyle. Age Concern offers a range of exercise classes for older people, including chair-based exercise for those who have limited ability. Joyce (64) came out of hospital after an operation and was nervous about getting mobile again. She wanted to improve her health and fitness so that she could play with her grandchildren. Robin, the project leader gave her advice about diet and exercise. He also gave her a pedometer. As you may know we are supposed to do 10,000 steps a day to improve our fitness. Janet enjoyed walking. When she was wearing the pedometer, she was determined to improve the number of steps she took, as Robin gave her a daily chart on which to record the number of steps she took each day. She found she lost weight and felt more energetic.

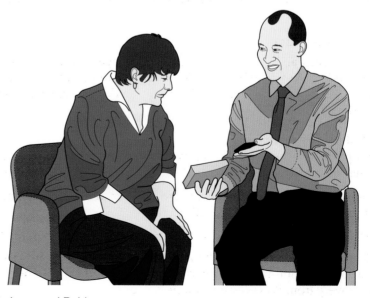

Figure 4.31 Joyce and Robin

Why did Joyce decide to improve her fitness?

Because she was motivated in her approach to exercise she was happy to do the walking.

Very often it is difficult to motivate people. They say they don't have time.

Some people prefer group activities, others prefer to exercise on their own.

In one London borough various activities have been developed for a range of ages and abilities as part of the health and well-being programme.

These are some of the activities they do:

- Stay Active Everyday is a programme for adults living in the borough who are over 50 years of age. The aim of the programme is to encourage people to stay fit and active by doing at least 30 minutes of exercise three times every week. Sports and activities to choose from include gym, table tennis, swimming, dancing and tai chi.
- Magpie Dance offers classes for adults with learning disabilities and their support workers. Classes are designed to help mobility, self-confidence and team working.
- Sports sessions: MENCAP are offering regular sports sessions including netball, basket ball and aerobics.
- The Parkinson's Disease society offers physio and exercise classes.

Preventing ill health

The public health programmes we have discussed are aimed at preventing ill-health through exercise, diet and lifestyle changes. Not all ill-health can be prevented. In Chapter 2 we discussed how immunisation against disease can be effective against childhood illnesses.

Primary prevention

This aims to prevent the onset of disease. Immunisation would be an example of primary prevention. Giving up smoking would reduce a person's chance of lung disease.

Secondary prevention

This aims to detect and cure a disease at an early stage. Screening for cancer of the breast and cervix would be examples of secondary prevention. Diabetes is an example where early diagnosis and control can delay or prevent many of the complications of diabetes.

Improving fitness levels

Many people believe that if they improve their fitness levels they will keep healthy. Do you remember the definition of health from the World Health Organisation?

WHO defines health as a 'state of complete physical, mental and social well-being and not merely the absence of infirmity'.

However, we all have ideas about what to be healthy means to us as individuals.

Being fit may help you feel good about yourself and improve your sense of mental well-being, but it cannot guard against disease. It can also help you have a speedy recovery from illness or operations.

Improving life expectancy

Life expectancy has increased in the UK in the last 20 years.

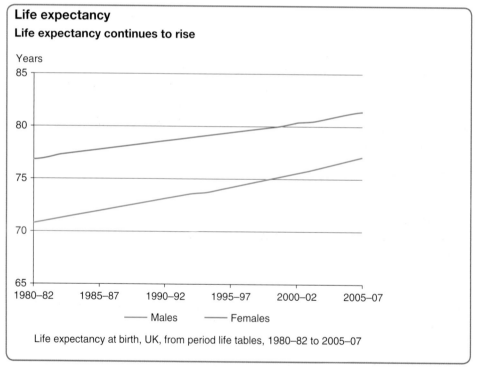

Life expectancy
Life expectancy continues to rise

Life expectancy at birth, UK, from period life tables, 1980–82 to 2005–07

Table 4.5 Life expectancy

Source: ONS online

In 2008 life expectancy at birth in the UK, has reached its highest level on record for both males and females. A newborn baby boy could expect to live 77.2 years and a newborn baby girl could live until 81.5 years if mortality rates remain the same as they were in 2005–07. Within the UK, England has the highest life expectancy at birth, while Scotland has the lowest. However, life expectancy rates differ among different social class groups and different ethnic groups.

The approaches used in health promotion

There are four different approaches to health promotion.

1. Medical or preventive: this approach aims to prevent disease.
2. Behaviour change/Educational: these approaches are to do with making sure people are well-informed and able to make healthy choices about their lifestyle.
3. Empowerment: this approach is to do with helping people acquire the skills and confidence to take greater control over their health.
4. Social change: this approach is to change policies and society in order to help all people make healthy choices.

Government health targets

The government sets health targets aimed at improving the health of the whole population. Areas of concern are identified and then specific targets are set. Although national targets are set, different areas of the UK differ in their populations and in their morbidity and mortality rates.

Examples of health improvement targets for 2008 (Scottish Health Improvement Targets for 2008).

- reduce mortality from coronary heart disease among the under 75s in deprived areas
- 80% of all 3–5 year-old-children to be registered with an NHS dentist
- achieve agreed completion rates for child healthy weight intervention programme by 2010/11
- reduce suicide rate between 2002 and 2013 by 20%
- through smoking cessation services, support 8% of smoking population in successfully quitting over the period 2008/9–2010/11
- increase the proportion of newborn children exclusively breastfed at 6–8 weeks from 26.6% in 2006/07 to 33.3% in 2010/11.

ACTIVITY

Read through the targets. Do you think they are realistic? Is it possible for people in deprived areas to change their lifestyles and diet so they may be more healthy?

We know there is a shortage of NHS dentists and to cope with this, the government has recruited dentists from overseas. People who are well-off are able to afford to pay for a private dentist, but people in deprived areas will not be able to afford this.

Statistics show that the suicide rate is highest among Social Class 4 (the lower socio-economic level) and young men are more likely to commit suicide. It would seem that suicide is related to socio-economic factors that are difficult to change.

Studies have also shown that many people who continue to smoke are from lower socio-economic levels and they find the only way they can cope is to smoke, as a means of being able to relax.

Mothers from lower socio-economic levels are less likely to continue to breast feed because they need to get back to work to support the family.

In all these examples, we can see that the social change approach to health promotion and health improvement needs to change society, so that people are financially supported in order that they can access a healthier lifestyle and diet.

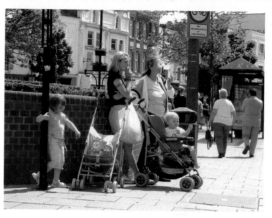

Figure 4.32 Cigarettes help some people cope with stress

In a London borough the National Health Improvement Targets have been analysed by the Public Health Strategy Group. This steering group works in partnership with the local authority, the NHS Trusts, schools, voluntary sector organisations and other services in the local area

The PHSG has worked in partnership to identify the issues that are most relevant to the local area. They have done this by looking at mortality and morbidity rates in the area; examining statistics related to health issues, and asking the local people what are their main concerns.

(See Chapter 2 on needs assessment page 76.)

Through this process four inequalities have been chosen in the first part of the 5-year programme in improving health in the area:

- reducing the mortality rate from all circulatory disease at ages under 75
- increasing adult participation in sport
- reducing obesity among primary school children in the reception year
- encouraging children to walk or cycle to school (reducing pollution and improving level of exercise taken)

Every three months the Public Health Steering Group reports back on the progress made on these targets.

The London borough has a population that is older than the London average so this is also taken into account when deciding upon targets. The Strategic Needs Assessment (see page 77) identified key targets for social services. These targets look at particular age groups and other groups in the population.

Priority	Description of indicator
Adult health and well-being	Reduce mortality rate from all circulatory disease at ages under 75
Adult health and well-being	Social care clients receiving social care support will be increased
Adult health and well-being	Carers will receive needs assessment and a specific carers service or advice and information
Tackling exclusion and promoting equality	Adults with learning disabilities will move from long-term hospital into the community

Table 4.5 Targets for social services

As you can see from the table, the local area committee has focused on issues that are relevant to their area when deciding what issues are important in the community. Many carers do not receive an assessment, partly because they are not identified.

Whenever a health and well-being plan is developed, you need to collect information about the current situation, so that you can track the progress being made. The information you start with is called the base line, and then progress is measured from this initial starting point.

There are 20 priorities for children and young people in this borough and these are mainly about children in care receiving support, education and moving into suitable training or employment. As we have seen in Chapter 1, training and education are an important factor in personal development and on health and well-being.

All local councils are concerned about 'sustainable living'. This means that environment conditions are seen to be important for health and well-being, and best use is made of the facilities in the area.

These are some of the priorities in the Sustainable Living part of the Health and Well-being plan.

Priority	Indicator description
Stronger communities	Participation for all age groups in sport
Environmental sustainability	Reduce CO_2 emissions in the area
Environmental sustainability	Improved local biodiversity – active management of local sites
Environmental sustainability	Reduction in car use taking children to school

Table 4.6 Priorities for sustainable living

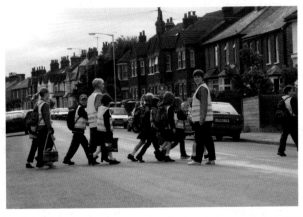

Figure 4.33 'Walk to school days' are one way of reducing the use of cars to take children to school.

ACTIVITY

In your area there should be a similar Public Health Plan. This should be on the website of the local authority where you live. A council website is a very useful source of information, as it will tell you about all the services that are provided as well as the health and social care targets in the area.

How health professionals support individuals to change health-related behaviour

Diagnosis

In order to be able to diagnose a disease or illness, professionals have to be able to recognise the signs and symptoms that are relevant. In the 1950s many diagnoses were made by detailed physical examination of the patients; taking their medical history, asking them about the symptoms they had, for how long etc.; looking at the patient for outward signs – like sweating, a flushed or pale face and other signs. There were limited tests to help the doctor diagnose – some simple blood and urine tests and X-rays.

Nowadays, there is a battery of tests the doctor or nurse can order for the patients. MRI scans and other investigations have made diagnosis much easier than in the past.

We see on page 237 below, that once a diagnosis is made, treatment will be discussed with the patient.

In the case of asthma (see pages 240–1) the care giver will need to give advice on a healthy life style to prevent the condition becoming out of control.

In the case of other chest disease – such as Chronic Obstructive Pulmonary Disease (COPD) – it may be difficult for the care giver to influence behaviour change in adults who have smoked all their lives and may have poor respiratory function as a result.

> **KEY TERM**
>
> **MRI scans-magnetic resonance imaging** – These are used to diagnose a range of problems but are particularly useful when diagnosing malfunctions of the brain and spinal cord.

> **CASE STUDY 15**
>
> **John is 45**
>
> John is 45 and he has always been a heavy smoker. When he was diagnosed with COPD he found it very difficult to give up smoking. When he finally gave up, he put on a lot of weight and became very depressed. He went to a self-help group that had been set up locally for people with COPD. This group was called Breathe Easy. The group had speakers to give them advice about lifestyle. The thing that John found most helpful was to meet other people in the same boat. He became very interested in how breathing exercises could be helpful. He went on some training courses and came back and led the group in exercises at each meeting. He felt much better as he was doing something he had chosen to do, rather than being told to do something.

Monitoring progress

As described on page 237, once a diagnosis is made, and treatment is started, it is necessary to monitor the progress that the service user is making:

- Is the patient having a reaction to any of the medication?
- Could the dosage of a drug be reduced?
- Is the patient able to lead an independent life?
- Are blood tests, blood pressure or other tests normal, or is there still cause for concern?

Monitoring can be done by a range of practitioners.

Pharmacists are becoming more involved in patient care; they may advise on drug issues; they may take blood pressures of patients on hypertension medication. Nurses and doctors monitor their patients.

EXAMPLE 1

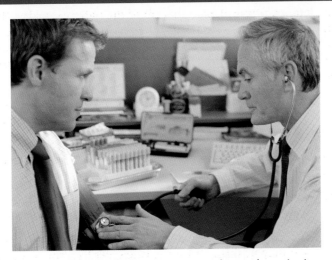

Figure 4.34 Monitoring blood pressure is very important

Robert is 42. He has put on weight in the last year. He saw his GP for a health check for his firm. His GP found Robert's blood pressure was rather high and he was several kilos overweight. Because Robert's mother had diabetes and a heart condition, the doctor tested Robert's urine. He sent Robert to the hospital for blood tests and an ECG to test his heart function. He gave Robert a diet sheet and told him to reduce his intake of beer and fats. When Robert next saw the doctor, he was told that his heart was healthy and all his other tests were normal; he had no trace of diabetes and his cholesterol levels were low. Robert attended the surgery every 6 weeks, but his blood pressure was still high, so in the end he was put on some tablets for his blood pressure. Robert was also asked by his GP to buy a BP machine from the pharmacy so that he could monitor his blood pressure himself and record it in-between each visit.

DISCUSSION

What do you think of the way the GP interacted with Robert? Can you think of any problems? Not everyone can afford to buy their own blood pressure monitor. However, giving Robert the opportunity to monitor himself makes him feel part of the process.

Health planning

It is very difficult to draw up a health plan with some patients and for them to follow it. The plan needs to be realistic. If the plan includes exercising, it is important that the patient chooses the exercise they enjoy, if the plan is to be successful. Plans have to fit into people's lives – not the other way round. When devising a plan, it is important to look at the lifestyle of the person and to see how any planned change can fit into their daily routine.

Advice and counselling

CASE STUDY 13 – Lucy

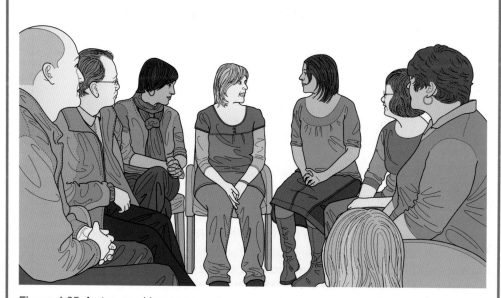

Figure 4.35 A stop smoking group

Norma

Norma has always been a heavy smoker. Her health has suffered as a result. She was diagnosed with osteoporosis and she has decided she must make an effort to stop 'the fags', as she calls them. Her GP recommended that she should go to the smoking cessation support group, which meets every week in the local clinic. She was nervous about going but felt she had nothing to lose. The group was quite small and included all ages; there were more women than men. The health advisor started off the session, introducing herself and the others in the groups introduced them selves. They were all asked why they had decided to give up smoking. Reasons given were the cost of the cigarettes, as well as health reasons. Then Tina, the advisor, asked them why they found it hard to give up. Norma found this very interesting as everyone had a different reason – from helping them cope with stress to anxiety about putting on weight. At the end of the session the advisor gave them details of other support that they could use to help them give up smoking. They could phone up a helpline for support; they could be 'health buddies' to each other so they could phone or text each other if things were difficult. Tina, the health advisor said she could also refer people for counselling, as very often people had problems and used smoking as a way of dealing with these difficulties and the counsellor may be able to help them see their problems differently and this could help them give up.

Evaluating progress against targets

We have seen how people's health targets are monitored earlier in this chapter. Evaluation means that instead of just noting the reduction in Norma's smoking, the change is discussed with the service user. Is this enough progress for the time being? Do we need to review the targets that were set? Does the person need additional help to meet the target that has been set?

How effective promotion and support for health improvements is built upon through the careful implementation of care values

A London borough has outlined the seven outcomes endorsed for the users of Adult Social Services.

They are as follows:

- improved health and emotional well-being
- improved quality of life
- making a positive contribution (to the community)
- choice and control
- freedom from discrimination
- economic well-being
- personal dignity.

We can see that these outcomes reflect many of the care values we have discussed in Chapter 2 and elsewhere.

Promotion of choice

Health improvement can only come about if everyone is working together. That means the council, the health services, early years services and the people themselves. No one likes to be told what to eat, what to do, or how to spend their money when they go to the supermarket. If health promotion programmes are to be effective they need to encourage people to make the healthy choices.

Respecting identity and culture

In a multi-cultural society like the UK, a range of cultural views about health and illness exist at any one time. For example, the traditional Chinese medicine is based on the idea of Yin and Yang– female and male, hot and cold – which is applied to symptoms, diets and treatments such as acupuncture and Chinese herbal medicine. Alternative practitioners offer therapies based on these cultural views of health and disease. Health practitioners are encouraged to look at the whole person (rather than the disease) and to treat each person as an individual.

Practitioners are developing approaches where discussion takes place between the patient and the doctor, or other practitioner, so that treatment or a care plan develops as a result of this collaboration.

Empowerment

As we have seen in this chapter, empowering patients and clients in health and social care can mean giving people the skills and knowledge so that they can feel part of the planning of their care. The Expert Patient Programme (2001) was developed by the Department of Health. The idea behind this programme was that patients with chronic conditions – such as arthritis, asthma and diabetes – could manage their own care. Some user-led self-management training programmes have been developed for people with chronic conditions. The Department of Health argues that people living with these chronic conditions often have a lot of knowledge about their condition and some PCTs have developed sessions when 'expert patients', who have received training, tell people with the same disease how they manage their condition.

There is more about the Expert Patient Programme on www.expertpatients.nhs.uk

Promoting independence

We have seen in Chapter 2 that promoting independence is a key core value in social care. Professionals need to support service users so that they can live independently and make the right health choices in their lives. This is closely related to empowerment.

CASE STUDY 17

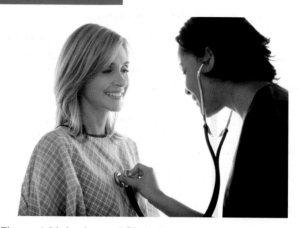

Figure 4.36 Lesley and Charlotte

Lesley is a nurse practitioner in a busy health centre. She specialises in looking after the asthma patients in the practice. This means that she is looking after patients that include babies, teenagers, adults and older people. She finds her job very demanding. When people are first diagnosed with asthma they can be very upset, or the parents of young children can be very anxious. She encourages these patients and explains carefully how asthma does not mean that life will change and you will not be able to do the things you have always done. Charlotte (28) was diagnosed with asthma when she came back from a holiday and she was breathless and had a bad cough. Charlotte could not believe it, but her peak flow was very low. Lesley listened to her chest and sent her for a chest x-ray. The x-ray showed Charlotte had a chest infection, which was treated using antibiotics, but she still had problems breathing, especially at night when her cough was worse. Charlotte was shown how to use the various inhalers. There was a blue one to open up the airways; an orange one which contained a steroid in a low dose and a green one, which was called a preventer that helped keep the airways in good condition. In the first few months Charlotte found it hard to cope with the idea she had asthma. She saw Lesley every week, or so, until things settled down. Now Charlotte feels confident about managing her asthma. She avoids things she knows make her asthma worse, like smoky rooms and bonfires. She goes swimming as she finds the warm damp atmosphere helps her chest.

(continued)

> **CASE STUDY 17– (continued)**
>
> Occasionally, she has to borrow a nebuliser from the surgery if she gets very wheezy or has a chest infection. She always makes sure she takes all her medication with her if she goes on holiday. She has a reserve supply of oral steroid pills she can take if her asthma is difficult to control. She sees Lesley once a year nowadays for a check up, when her peak flow is measured by a spirometer – a more sensitive device than a peak flow monitor. Charlotte feels confident she can manage.

We can see from this example that it is helpful for both the service user and the direct carer to encourage independence in people who can safely manage their conditions.

Respecting individual right to choice

Much of the recent guidance for the Department of Health is about promoting choice for patients. One of these initiatives in health was called Patient Choice, when patients who were going to be referred to a hospital for an operation such as hip or knee replacements, or other procedures, were asked to make a choice about the hospital they should go to. The GP surgery was supposed to offer a choice of several hospitals and the patients could choose. In practice, this has been difficult. Most people preferred to rely on the recommendation of their GP. The IT system that supported this programme had intermittent difficulties.

Many people have access to the Internet and, as we have seen in Chapter 2, reports on hospitals are available on the web, so patients are better informed about health matters nowadays, but it may still be difficult for them to make an informed choice.

Direct payments

In social care there have been several moves to encourage patient choice through the development of Direct Payments, when the patient is allocated a budget by social services and a care plan is worked out with the service user, their carer (if they have one) and the care manager. From 2010–2011 Social Services will have to operate a new system called Transforming Social Care, when service users will be assessed and given an amount of money in their personal budget to use as they wish. They could decide to spend it in trips to the pub – as a way of reducing social exclusion. Pilot areas have been trying out the new system. In one area, the male service user wanted to buy a dog with his budget and this was seen as a good way of improving his health by increasing his activity, and also on a social level by having the companionship of a pet.

The main groups of service users that will have personal budgets are likely to be:

- people with physical disabilities
- people with learning disabilities
- people with mental health problems.

However, some service providers are anxious about how the system will operate. Some people will not want to have the bother of managing personal budgets; other service providers are anxious about how the money will be used – as this money is public money paid for by tax payers.

Local social services are developing systems so that the new process will work effectively, giving people more choice and giving support to those who do not want to have the responsibility for their own budget.

In this chapter we have seen that the care values we have discussed through this book are still relevant to all aspects of health improvement.

GLOSSARY

Absolute poverty – a lack of resources sufficient to maintain a healthy existence

Abuse – treating people badly, either physically or emotionally

Amniocentesis – a test in which some of the amniotic fluid that surrounds the baby in the womb is removed to test for genetic disorders

Asthma – disease in which there is narrowing of the airways, leading to wheezing, coughing, tightness of the chest and shortness of breath

Blood glucose test – measurement of glucose level in blood

Blood pressure – the pressure at which blood flows through the circulatory system

Body mass index (BMI) – a simple assessment of body mass.

$$BMI = \frac{body\ mass/kg}{(height/m)^2}$$

Bronchitis – disease in which the small airways are blocked and damaged, leading to a severe cough producing large quantities of phlegm (a mix of mucus, bacteria and white blood cells)

Carcinogen – cancer causing chemical (e.g. in tar found in cigarettes)

Cardiovascular diseases – conditions that affect the heart and circulation

Cholesterol – a fat that occurs naturally in the body; can build up in arteries, causing heart disease

Chorionic villus sampling (CVS) – a test in which some of the placenta is removed to test for genetic disorders in the baby

Chronic condition – a disease of long duration involving very slow changes. It often starts very gradually

Cohabitation – a couple living together who are not married or in a civil partnership

Culture – shared values based on beliefs, practice, dress, language, diet and religion

Discrimination – the unfair treatment of a person, or group, because of a negative view of some, or all, of their characteristics (could be based on ethnicity, gender or age)

Disease – a specific condition of ill health, identified as an actual change on the surface or inside some part of the body (Compare with Illness)

DNA (deoxyribonucleic acid) – the molecule that forms the genetic material

Emotional health – concerned with being able to express feelings such as fear, joy, grief, frustration and anger. It also includes the ability to cope with anxiety, stress, and depression

Emotional health – concerned with the ability to recognise emotions such as fear, joy, grief, frustration and anger, and to express such emotions appropriately

GLOSSARY – (continued)

Emphysema – disease in which there is breakdown of air sacs in the lungs, leading to wheezing and shortness of breath.

Ethnicity – a shared identity that comes from a common culture, religion or tradition

Ethnicity – a shared identity which comes from a common culture, religion or tradition

Gender – the psychological and social development of male and female roles in a society

Holistic – looking at the whole system rather than just concentrating on individual components

Homophobia – fear and hatred of homosexuals

Ideal self – the type of person you would most like to be

Identity – self image; how you see yourself and what you know about yourself

Illness – the subjective state of feeling unwell (i.e. how people feel). (Compare with Disease and Sickness)

Income – the sum of all earnings of a household or individual in a given period of time

Intellectual health – concerned with the ability to think clearly and rationally

Intellectual health – this is concerned with the ability to think clearly and rationally. It is closely linked to emotional and social health.

Liver function test (LFT) – measure of chemicals in blood made by liver

Material possessions – the things a person owns

Menopause – when women stop menstruating

Mutation – an unpredictable change in genetic material.

Nicotine – drug in tobacco that causes addiction and increases heart rate and blood pressure

Nuclear family – family consisting of one woman and one man with dependent children

Obesity – the excessive deposit of fat under the skin.

Objective – based on facts, not personal feelings or opinions

Peak flow – a measure of how fast you can blow air out of your lungs.

Physical health – concerned with the physical functioning of the body. It is the easiest aspect of health to measure.

Physical health – concerned with the physical functioning of the body

Poverty – lack of resources helping you to be healthy

Primary relationship – close relationship based on kinship, marriage, adoption, friendship or blood ties

Pulse – regular pulsation in blood flow through arteries

Recovery pulse rate – time taken for pulse to return to normal rate after exercise

Redundancy – when work or a job no longer exists for the worker who is then made unemployed

GLOSSARY – (continued)

Relative poverty – a lack of resources (income) sufficient to achieve a standard of living considered acceptable in a society

Respiratory diseases – conditions that affect breathing, such as asthma and bronchitis

Role model – an example of behaviour or achieved status in society that is seen as good

Rural area – a sparsely populated area; as well as agricultural areas, rural areas include 'honey pot' villages that rely heavily on tourism, urban fringe commuter villages and former coal-mining communities

Screening – a simple test carried out on a large number of apparently healthy people to separate those who probably have a certain disease from those who do not.

Secondary relationship – more distant or formal relationship that may be short term

Self-concept – how you see yourself as a separate individual

Self-esteem – the value you place on yourself

Self-fulfilling prophecy – a belief that things turn out as you predict because people behave in such a way as to bring about the prediction- usually to do with behaviour

Self-image (identity) – how you see yourself and what you know about yourself

Sibling – brother or sister

Sickness – reported illness; involves being treated by a professional and becoming a medical statistic

Social exclusion – when an individual is prevented from taking part in any of the key economic, social and political activities in the society in which they live

Social health – concerned with the ability to relate to others and to form relationships with other people

Social health – this is concerned with the ability to relate to others and to form relationships

Social role – the way you behave in certain situations, such as a student, nurse, etc

Socialisation – the way you learn as a child how to fit into society using the social skills and values of that society

Socio-economic group – category people are put in depending on their social class, wealth and income and education

Sphygmomanometer – equipment used for measuring blood pressure

Status – your social position related to others so may be high or low; linked to factors such as wealth, income, social class, job, age and appearance

Stereotype – a simplified general image about a particular group of people, e.g. 'they all do that'

Stress – the inability to cope with change

Subjective – based on an individual's point of view

Urban area – town or city

GLOSSARY – (continued)

Vaccine – a preparation given to a person to stimulate their white blood cells to produce antibodies, so that they will not develop a disease when they come in contact with the bacteria or virus that causes it.

Waist/hip ratio

$$= \frac{\text{Waist measurement}}{\text{Hip measurement}}$$

Wealth – the extent of an individual's or household's possessions and resources

Working relationship – relationship based in working environment that is more distant or formal

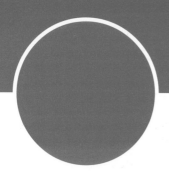

INDEX